# TREATING ATTACHMENT DISORDERS

AST
TRUST
MATION

# Treating Attachment Disorders
## From Theory to Therapy

KARL HEINZ BRISCH

*Translated by Kenneth Kronenberg*
*Foreword by Lotte Köhler*
*Afterword by Inge Bretherton*

THE GUILFORD PRESS
New York    London

German edition published as *Bindungsstörungen:*
*Von der Bindungstheorie zur Therapie*
Klett-Cotta
© 1999 J. G. Cotta'sche Buchhandlung Nachfolger GmbH
Stuttgart


English edition © 2002 The Guilford Press
A Division of Guilford Publications, Inc.
72 Spring Street, New York, NY 10012
www.guilford.com

Printed in the United States of America

This book is printed on acid-free paper.

Last digit is print number:  9  8  7  6  5  4  3  2

**Library of Congress Cataloging-in-Publication Data**

Brisch, Karl Heinz.
    [Bindungsstorungen. English]
    Treating attachment disorders : from theory to therapy / by Karl Heinz
Brisch.
        p.   cm.
Includes bibliographical references and index.
    ISBN 1-57230-681-5
  1. Attachment disorder in children. I. Title.
    RJ507.A77 B7513 2002
    618.92′89—dc21                                    2002004450

*I dedicate this book to my children,*
*Verena, Nicola, and Jonathan,*
*and to my wife, Lizzy*

*Through them I learned much about attachment*

Attachment theory regards the propensity to make intimate emotional bonds to particular individuals as a basic component of human nature, already present in germinal form in the neonate and continuing through adult life in to old age. During infancy and childhood bonds are with parents (or parent substitutes) who are looked to for protection, comfort, and support. During healthy adolescence and adult life these bonds persist, but are complemented by new bonds, commonly of a heterosexual nature. Although food and sex sometimes play important roles in attachment relationships, the relationship exists in its own right and has a key survival function of its own, namely protection.

—JOHN BOWLBY (1988, pp. 120–121)

# About the Author

**Karl Heinz Brisch, MD,** is a child and adolescent psychiatrist and psychotherapist, as well as an adult psychiatrist and neurologist; a training psychoanalyst at the Psychoanalytic Institute; and head of the Department of Pediatric Psychosomatic Medicine and Psychotherapy at the Children's Hospital at the Ludwig-Maximilians-University of Munich, Germany. Dr. Brisch's primary research is in the development of infants and children with high-risk conditions and the development of attachment and its disorders. He has led longitudinal research projects on attachment disturbances and early psychotherapeutic interventions. He is also a member of the World Association of Infant Mental Health and of the Society for Research in Child Development.

~

# Contents

ix

# Acknowledgments
# to the English Edition

I owe a debt of gratitude to many persons, without whose assistance this English-language edition would never have seen the light of day. I was very fortunate that Inge Bretherton and Anni Bergmann picked up the newly published German edition while at a conference in Germany, and after reading it encouraged me to have it translated into English. Dr. Knappe of the German publishing house Klett-Cotta sought out financing for such a translation. Funding from the German cultural agency Inter-Nationes made the translation possible. I thank Seymour Weingarten of The Guilford Press for his engaged support and continuing interest. He made certain that the right people undertook the work, and that it was completed in good time. I found a most competent and resourceful translator in Kenneth Kronenberg, who shared with me his editorial consultant, Eve Golden, MD. He kept in steady contact with me during the translation process, and I am grateful to him for his sensitivity and hard work. I owe special thanks to Inge Bretherton. She was indefatigable in reading and commenting on the various manuscript drafts that landed in her in-box. In particular, the English version was much improved by her comments on the theoretical section and by her citation of papers and studies that appeared after publication of the German edition.

With all my heart I thank my wife, Lizzy, and my children, Verena, Nicola, and Jonathan, who, I'm afraid, often had to make do with less than my full attention while I was working on the translation. I am deeply grateful for their understanding and encouragement.

# Acknowledgments
## to the German Edition

I owe a debt of thanks to many people, without whose help this book could never have been written.

I particularly wish to thank Lotte Köhler, who encouraged me from the very beginning to write this book, and motivated me to produce it. She read the manuscript in many versions and offered discerning and useful criticism and advice. She has been, so to speak, my "secure base" in this undertaking.

I thank Karin Grossmann for her helpful comments on the theoretical section and for her ideas on grounding the cases in attachment theory.

My colleague Anna Buchheim contributed her knowledge of attachment theory and attachment research to our working group. Over the past several years this has encouraged much discussion in many ways, and the results are integrated into the book also. I thank her, as well as my colleagues Gesine Schmücker, Brigitte Köhntop, Susanne Betzler, Doro Munz, Kristin Bemmerer-Mayer, Gerhart Mahler, Ute Barth, and Irina Zimmer, for combing through the manuscript.

I thank Horst Kächele for his critical examination of the theoretical section; he alerted me to some important discrepancies and made further suggestions.

Thanks also to pediatrician Walter Teller, who improved the readability of the text and helped make it comprehensible to non-psychotherapists.

Thanks too to my colleagues and friends, especially Johannes Brehm, Hans Hopf, Annegret Rein, and Christoph Walker, for reading the manuscript and for helpful suggestions and friendly support.

Special thanks to my secretary, Birgit Vogel, who with great dedication has done the typing from the very beginning of the project. Without her, this book would never have been produced in such a short time.

I thank my wife, Lizzy, without whose emotional support and critical feedback I would not have been able to get through this strenuous period nearly as well as I did. I thank my children, who had to go without my attention during this time, for their understanding. As my daughter justly remarked, there should have been a chapter in this book about the "disorders" to attachment relationships that can occur within the family when the father is writing a book.

I also owe special thanks to Mathilde Fischer of Klett-Cotta Verlag, whose suggestion gave initial impetus to this book. During the entire period of its writing, she followed the process as an encouraging reader and made sure that the publisher would produce the book as quickly as possible.

I also wish to take this opportunity to thank all of my patients and their parents, whose consent to the publication of their cases provided the essential basis for this book.

# Foreword

## Lotte Köhler

In the 1950s the English psychoanalyst John Bowlby was asked to fulfill two missions: to produce a report for the World Health Organization (WHO) on the psychological state of parents and children left homeless by the war, and to set up a child psychotherapy department at London's Tavistock Clinic. The knowledge he gained in the doing led him to a new theory—attachment theory—that diverged from the metatheory of psychoanalysis.

Attachment theory holds that human beings, in common with a number of other life forms, possess a biologically based *attachment system* that is activated as soon as an external or internal danger appears. If one's own resources are not sufficient to eliminate the danger, the phenomenon called *attachment behavior* is triggered: a small child turns to a familiar person—his mother or father, for example—toward whom he has built a very specific "attachment." His feelings, expectations, and behavioral strategies are directed toward this attachment relationship, which develops out of his experiences with these most important caregivers. Although the attachment pattern that takes shape as a result of his adaptation to them during the first years of life may change over the course of time, in most cases its basic structure remains relatively constant.

This person who furnishes protection and care is of life-preserving importance to the dependent human newborn and infant, and so, therefore, is the infant's attachment to this person. But the need for a "safe haven"—a reliable attachment figure who furnishes protection and help in dangerous situations—remains throughout life. In adults too, danger activates the attachment system that was formed during early childhood and triggers protection-seeking attachment behavior.

When Bowlby presented these ideas to his colleagues in London during the 1960s, he met with bitter resistance from psychoanalysts, because his theory was based not on current Freudian metapsychology and drive theory, but on cybernetic and systems models. Bowlby was also accused of simply explaining behavior and not addressing the "inner reality" that psychoanalysts address. In consequence of this dispute, psychoanalysis and attachment theory went their separate ways.

Bowlby's attachment theory was accepted by and integrated into academic developmental psychology, however, as other developmentalists devised methods that produced objective and reproducible information about attachment patterns and behavior. In particular, the "Strange Situation" procedure, developed by Bowlby's colleague Mary Ainsworth for 12-month-olds, has become a standard instrument for assessing the quality of attachment in infancy.

An important qualitative leap occurred when Mary Main and her colleagues developed methods for examining and evaluating attachment in adults with the Adult Attachment Interview. These methods make it possible to conclude with some certainty that the mother's *"state of mind" with respect to attachment* defines how she relates to the child. The Adult Attachment Interview (AAI) conducted with a still-pregnant mother enabled accurate prediction of the attachment pattern that the as yet unborn child would exhibit toward the mother at 1 year. This suggested that the mother's internal representations of attachment relationships influenced her subsequent interactions with her child and hence the child's attachment patterns to her. These findings provided a potential basis for a reconciliation between attachment theory and psychoanalysis.

*This is where we stand now.*

Before looking at the application of attachment theory to clinical practice, we need to take a closer look at the fundamental methodological presuppositions of psychoanalysis and of attachment theory. These explain in part why psychoanalysis and attachment theory pursued different paths for so long.

Psychoanalytic understanding is based on material gained in treatment from free association and from transference and countertransference phenomena. Analyst and patient together create a *reconstruction* of the patient's developmental history, establishing in this way what conditions led to the development of his psychological disorder. This process involves not just attachment behavior but the entire personality as it manifests itself in the course of intensive collaborative work between patient and therapist over a long period of time. Furthermore, psychoanalytic understanding derives primarily from the presentations of individual patients.

By contrast, attachment research relies on studies of more targeted and therefore more limited questions. Data are obtained from children of specific age groups, by both quantitative and qualitative methods, which are then analyzed statistically. Groups of parent–child dyads can be studied, in some cases from before birth all the way to adulthood, using reliable observational instruments. Such systematic longitudinal studies, which are very rare in psychoanalysis, confirm the correctness of Bowlby's position, as does modern infant research in general: namely, that the influence of external reality on the formation of internal reality must not be neglected. Although attachment studies have the advantage of reproducibility, they, unlike the psychoanalytic method, apprehend only certain details of development or personality. Brisch repeatedly stresses that attachment theory is characterized by a "partial view"; it does not claim to shed light on all aspects of human personality.

The study and spread of attachment theory has led to a vast published literature and a great deal of important information about the various attachment patterns and behavioral styles, the conditions under which they arise, and their further development over the life cycle. This enables us to make statements about which attachment patterns are adaptive or maladaptive in the conditions of any contemporary society, and which ones should in fact be seen as pathogenic; there are attachment patterns that may be life-preserving in times of war and pestilence but that prove harmful in times of peace and prosperity.

Now, a situation in which a patient is seeking help from a physician or therapist represents precisely the sort of trigger that activates the attachment system. Therefore it seems clear that knowledge of attachment patterns, and the conditions under which they arise, is important to all health professionals. It facilitates both the good doctor–patient relationships that are essential to successful treatment and comprehension and management of the therapeutic process as a whole.

Psychoanalysis has only recently accepted the importance of attachment theory, and there is little literature examining the application of attachment theory to clinical practice from the psychoanalytic perspective.[1]

This book by Karl Heinz Brisch fills that gap. Brisch gives us a short overview of John Bowlby's personal development and a history of the development of attachment theory, presents the methods and findings of attachment research, and familiarizes the reader with the various forms of "attachment disorders."

Finally, Brisch turns his attention to the psychoanalytic method of presenting individual cases, and illustrates the value of applying an attachment theory perspective by interpreting numerous case histories through the lens of attachment theory. The clinician and/or practitioner will find these helpful. Brisch focuses on aspects relevant to attachment. This can create the impression of a certain one-sidedness, but it is a didactic expedient to introduce the reader to an attachment perspective. Nonetheless, it should be noted that Brisch repeatedly stresses that attachment theory is capable of explaining only *part* of the whole personality, although that is a part of crucial importance to interpersonal relationships. Moreover, he discusses the therapeutic consequences a different perspective might have had in some cases. These comparisons allow the reader to consider the attachment perspective in context.

The case presentations are relevant for another much-discussed reason. Attachment patterns acquired in early childhood are believed to be stored as what is called "procedural memory": as unconscious patterns of behavior and experience. In the course of development, however, they may become partially explicit and therefore accessible to reflection. For this reason, attachment problems may offer a particularly productive entry point, allowing the therapist to broach attachment issues that are accessible to consciousness, along with the new experiences resulting from transference. This approach offers the potential for changing unconscious procedural working models. How this may happen and how this might be conceptualized is right now being considered and discussed by "the Process of Change Study Group."[2]

At University Hospitals—formerly in Ulm and more recently in Munich—Brisch conducts attachment research and practices clinic-based psychoanalysis. He is at home in both fields. With his broad medical training in psychiatry, neurology, child and adolescent psychiatry, and psychopharmacology, he has been able to build collaborative projects with representatives of the allied medical disciplines as well as with social workers, and among school personnel. He has shown them the possibilities of attachment-oriented intervention, thus sharpening their ability to spot problem cases, who are in turn referred to him.

This book makes clear just how fruitful a collaboration between therapists trained in attachment theory and the above-mentioned disciplines can be. This is true especially for gynecologists and pediatricians, but it applies to all members of the health and caring professions, even for those employed by health insurance companies. The case descriptions underscore, among other things, how expensive medical tests, diagnostic procedures, interventions, and treatments may be avoided in cases in which unresolved attachment problems have led to physical illnesses and behaviors that endanger health—accident-proneness is one example. The book explains to the reader how to understand such connections and what clues should awaken suspicion of an underlying attachment disorder.

In the final chapter of the book, Brisch presents his ideas about how attachment theory might be fruitfully applied in the areas of prevention, pedagogy, and family and group therapy. Even if only a few of the proposals in this book become reality, that in itself will be welcome progress.

# Preface

I clearly remember reading Bowlby's trilogy on attachment, separation, and loss during my psychoanalytic training, and wrestling with his theories about the development of attachment. But I did not know then how I could translate these stimulating theories into my psychotherapeutic practice, and attachment theory was absent from the case seminars I attended. Bowlby's work slid into the background, and I only rediscovered it during my medical training in psychiatry and in child and adolescent psychiatry. Many case histories showed me how important experiences of separation and loss apparently played a role in the development of my patients' illnesses. One way or another, attachment, separation, and autonomy found their way into each treatment, especially in child and adolescent psychiatry.

When I became director of outpatient care in child and adolescent psychiatry and psychotherapy at the University Hospital in Ulm, I was consulted about the psychotherapeutic treatment of parents whose premature newborns had been cared for in the neonatology department at the University Children's Clinic in Ulm. I had studied neonatology during my pediatric training, but that had been many years back, and I found it hard to believe how such extremely tiny premature newborns could even survive.

In the course of many discussions with the parents of premature babies, it became clear that they were confronted with an emotional crisis that I designate the "trauma of prematurity." These parents were grieving the loss of a pregnancy that had terminated too soon, and sometimes "out of the blue." They were not at all psychologically prepared for this. Despite unlimited visiting hours, I realized that it was very hard for these parents to form emotional bonds to such tiny newborns, when the beginning of life had occurred so unexpectedly and when the baby would have to be cared for in an incubator for weeks.

In collaboration with Frank Pohlandt, director of neonatology and pediatric intensive care at the University Hospital in Ulm, and his team, some very fruitful research developed out of this clinical situation. We studied the development of attachment in these tiny preemies, and later a further study of preventive psychotherapy for the parents was added.

I had the very good fortune to get to know Anna Buchheim during the design phase of these studies. She had been a student of Klaus Grossmann in Regensburg, and brought her knowledge of attachment theory with her to Ulm, beginning an intensive collaboration between clinical researchers on attachment in Ulm and the basic researchers Klaus and Karin Grossmann and their team.

Since then, we have expanded our clinical attachment research to include several aspects of the pre- and perinatal stages, thanks to our good working relationship with the University Women's Clinic in Ulm. We are now investigating such questions as how prenatal diagnosis and the problem of high-risk pregnancy with impending prematurity affect child development, the mother–child interaction, and the attachment of these children to their parents over time.

We key these basic research questions to the psychotherapeutic approach that we use with affected parents because, in our opinion, basic research and psychotherapeutic intervention must be closely linked if the situation of these parents is to improve.

Such linkage between psychotherapy research and clinical practice in a field that has been so neglected can only be accomplished through the cooperation of various disciplines—in this case, pediatrics, obstetrics, prenatal medicine, psychotherapy, psychosomatic medicine, and child and adolescent psychiatry. This exchange is only possible with the engagement of our colleagues in the working group and the openness and curiosity of colleagues in other clinics to the questions we pose.

Without my team's ability to create and maintain "attachments" across disciplinary lines, our activities would be doomed to failure.

Lack of space would have made it impossible for us to conduct our longitudinal studies of these at-risk children had it not been for Horst Kächele's far-sighted involvement and the financial support of the Köhler Foundation, Darmstadt, which gave us the research facilities that we needed.[1]

My research activities and my expanded understanding of attachment theory increasingly influenced my therapeutic procedures. I now understood the therapeutic process from a fresh perspective. I decided on a case approach because I am convinced that the practitioner can learn most from clinical examples. It should be noted, however, that we cannot generalize from case examples, and it was never my intent to do so.

In every description of a patient's history there is an ethical tension between the patient's right to privacy and confidentiality and the scientific interest in the particular case study. In some of our cases, patient consent could not be obtained—for example, because the person had moved and there was no forwarding address. In these cases, distinguishing characteristics were altered so that the individuals in question could not be recognized. However, the essential psychodynamic features were retained so that the development of the disorder and the course of treatment could be reconstructed.

Because attachment theory proposes that attachment is a lifelong developmental issue, I selected case studies from all age groups. I have structured the case histories consistently across the clinical spectrum so that readers can orient themselves more easily. Each case begins with my initial contact with the patient and the development of a particular therapeutic approach. This is followed by a description of the symptomatology and a biographical history. Specific reflections about attachment dynamics are derived from this base, which, for didactic reasons, focus specifically on the issue of attachment. However, other psychodynamic hypotheses and the techniques that derive from them may also at times be proposed. Sometimes I based my considerations on other theoretical backgrounds in order to encourage "contrarian thinking." Description of the course of treatment is followed by reflections on the therapy and additional information from the follow-up history, insofar as this is known.

This book deals with developments in a new area and represents a selective snapshot of the state of the research in this area, my own thinking, and my current perspective on the topic.

It is not my intention to found a new school of therapy with this book. It is much more to the point to imagine "attachment" as a fundamental variable in the psychotherapeutic process that might find a significant place in a general psychotherapeutic model that is not tied to a particular school.

~

# Introduction

In all psychotherapeutic work, whether it be with infants and their parents, with toddlers, children, or adolescents, or with adults, we confront the question of how to make sense of particular psychological symptoms. Today all psychotherapeutic schools, whatever their orientation, attribute to childhood a crucial role in the development of psychopathology (Kächele, Buchheim, & Brisch, 1999; Resch, 1996).

Psychoanalytic theories have derived from material gathered in the treatment of adult patients. The psychodynamic relationships that were discovered in the course of therapy pointed to stages of development in early childhood that were important for psychological development. The resulting theory has been called "adultopathomorphic," in that pathological symptoms in the adult were understood and interpreted as regressions to early childhood phases that were part of normal development. The concepts of "infantile regression" and "fixation to early developmental phases" played a very important role. In his early years, Freud still placed the importance of actual seductions in the foreground of his theory: actual early sexual abuses of children by those closest to them, including parents, were viewed by him as experiences traumatic to the child's psyche. He later distanced himself from this view and postulated that the sexual abuse recalled in adult analyses represented childhood fantasies. Freud never expressly explained why he changed his position, but he subsequently gave fantasy priority in psychic development.

1

Freud came to believe that the elaboration of fantasies was more important in the development of psychopathology than the actual experiences that his patients reported. He generally ascribed these reports to fantasy rather than to actual experience, and this is why psychoanalysis came to focus largely on the processing of unconscious fantasies in its therapeutic techniques, correspondingly neglecting the real experiences of its patients. It may be that Freud's theory of actual early childhood trauma resulting from sexual abuse was so explosive that he feared for his reputation as a scientist. His reputation was ambiguous at the time because his discovery of childhood sexuality, which challenged the bourgeois morality prevailing in Vienna at the end of the nineteenth century, had encountered skepticism and even outright rejection.

The Swiss psychiatrist Adolf Meyer (1957) developed a theory of actual trauma similar to Freud's early theory: a psychobiological concept based on Darwin, to which Bowlby later referred. Meyer felt that psychological development was importantly influenced by actual traumatic factors in the early childhood environment, not limited to sexual abuse. According to Meyer's theory, psychological illnesses result from the individual's failed attempt to react to actual psychosocial stresses. If the individual's attempt to adapt places too great a strain on him, symptoms of illness may occur. Varying capacities to adapt to later external stresses depend upon actual experiences encountered in early childhood during the child's first years in its family of origin and other important relationships.

London psychiatrist and psychoanalyst John Bowlby was consistently confronted by extreme actual early childhood trauma in the deeply disturbed children and adolescents whose life histories he studied. He realized that the effect of these traumatic events on the development of their personalities was significant, and he did not view the experiences reported by the children as products of fantasy. In looking for potential causes for the development of psychopathology in these children, he recognized that the experience of multiple early losses and separations from attachment figures took precedence over the other traumatic experiences that were reported. The moment of this clinical discovery, which was based on detailed case reports, may be seen as the birth hour of attachment theory. Nevertheless, the road from initial idea to full formulation was a long and arduous one for Bowlby. It must have been hard for him to imagine at first that his theory, initially so attacked, would find resonance in developmental psychology and be the impetus for much additional research.

This research has not been limited to London. It was conveyed by Bowlby's research team, in particular his Canadian colleague Mary Ainsworth, to many other countries, and attachment research is now taking place in the United States, Canada, Israel, Japan, Italy, the Netherlands, and Germany.

In Germany, research into attachment is closely associated with Klaus and Karin Grossmann, who worked previously in Bielefeld and are now professors of psychology at Regensburg University. This couple and their scientific team have gained worldwide respect for their prospective longitudinal studies of healthy full-term infants. One consistent focus of this research group has been the continuity of early interactional experiences and resulting attachment qualities from infancy to adolescence, and the transmission of attachment models from the adult generation to its children.

The basic research has become enormously diverse and has yielded such an abundance of data that an overview would burst the confines of this book.[1] For this reason, I will simply give an overview of the basic concepts of attachment research. Important findings for the clinical application of attachment research and for treatment based on attachment theory will also be discussed.

Bowlby himself was an engaged clinician who felt forced by his experiences in therapeutic practice to develop new formulations of accepted theoretical concepts. It is my intention to pick up on his clinical interests and make his theoretical knowledge available to practicing psychotherapists.

In Section I, I will give a short history of the development of attachment theory. After a brief summary of attachment theory itself, I will introduce important concepts that relate to it, especially regarding the significance of parental sensitivity, the quality of childhood attachment, and the representation of attachment in adults.

In connection with this, I will also discuss aspects of the transgenerational transmission of attachment models and the significance of risk and protective factors. In conclusion, I will explain the concepts of attachment and separation as put forward in other psychological theories and in various psychotherapeutic schools.

In Section II, I will present some theoretical aspects of a psychopathology of attachment—that is, of the concept of attachment disorder. In a historical overview I will show how today's diagnostic manuals, as well as some newer diagnostic systems specializing in infancy and early childhood, have begun to make use of attachment theory. Because previous classification systems have not afforded adequate ways of diagnosing attachment disorders, I will describe a more far-reaching and comprehensive classification of such disorders.

In Section III, I will formulate a theory for an attachment-oriented psychotherapeutic technique. In so doing I refer to psychotherapy research that sees the attachment relationship between therapist and patient[2] as an important factor in successful treatment.

Basic techniques and procedures of attachment-oriented treatment will be described. The focus will be on the initial contact between patient and therapist, the arrangement of the therapeutic setting, matters such as frequency and termination, and questions relating to attachment and autonomy in the therapeutic process.

In Section IV, I will describe case studies from clinical practice. For didactic reasons, the focus of my observations will be disorder of the attachment dynamic. I will pass over other possible interpretations in order to bring the issue of attachment disorder into relief. Of course, a patient's symptoms may be understood differently from other theoretical perspectives and then treated using a different technique.

In the case examples, I describe the development of attachment over the course of the patient's life from the time his parents decide on a pregnancy all the way to adulthood. This structure is based on the observation that attachment develops through a lifelong process that demands constant adaptation to new relationships and life situations.

In Section V, the last section, I will discuss the issue of prevention. I will present an approach to early attachment-oriented training, aimed at preventing later psychological problems, that may be offered to pregnant women and their partners as well as to parents of small children.

In view of the increasing problem of aggression and violence in preschools and schools, a program of early attachment-oriented prevention and counseling would seem an important undertaking. I will put forward guidelines for prevention in the school setting; these are consonant with current research on the connection between attachment and aggression.

I will make some observations regarding the extent to which an attachment-oriented approach might be transferable to and applicable in other settings, such as group or family psychotherapy.

I will conclude by discussing some questions that are still open and some perspectives on the continuing development of an attachment-oriented psychotherapy and the importance of attachment theory in psychotherapeutic training.

# Section I

~

# Attachment Theory and Its Basic Concepts

## HISTORICAL OVERVIEW

Like his father, a well-known surgeon, John Bowlby (1907–1990) initially studied medicine, completing his first course of studies at Cambridge with several distinctions. It is still not clear why, instead of continuing his training in London, he spent the next year teaching, first at a progressive boarding school, then at a school for maladjusted children. In her biography of Bowlby, Suzan van Dijken (1998) reports that during that time Bowlby read a book on developmental psychology that greatly impressed him. From a psychodynamic perspective, however, this is not an adequate explanation of Bowlby's interrupted studies. Bowlby came from a wealthy upper-middle-class English family. His father was very absorbed in his profession, and the children's contact with their mother was limited to a few set hours per day; they were cared for by a governess and several nursemaids. This rather distanced relationship with his mother, and the fact that he lost his most important attachment figure, his favorite nursemaid, at the age of 3, were important aspects of Bowlby's biography (Holmes, 1993). Given this childhood history, it is understandable that he might concern himself with issues of attachment, separation, and loss, both theoretically and in practice. From a psychodynamic perspective, one might hypothesize that Bowlby was stimulated by the above-mentioned book to reflect about his own

7

childhood. His involvement with a progressive school for children displaying unacceptable social behavior could also be understood as an attempt to learn about the dark side of society and his own psyche, neither of which he had yet examined. His temporarily dropping out of medical school might be viewed as a postadolescent phase, a period during which he disassociated himself in his ideas and interests from his family and from the path that had been prescribed for him. His involvement with adolescents and children was a crucial experience, both emotionally and substantively, and was to have a lasting effect on the later development of his theory.

His mentor at the school for maladjusted children advised Bowlby to go into child psychiatry, so when he went to the teaching hospital in London he had already decided to become a child psychiatrist. At that time he also began psychoanalytic training with a follower of Klein.

After finishing his medical studies, Bowlby sought training in the newly founded discipline of child psychiatry, and served at the London Child Guidance Clinic from 1936 until the beginning of World War II. He was also engaged in an examination of Melanie Klein's theories, concluding that she paid insufficient attention to environmental influences.

After the arrival of the Freuds in London in 1939, a long-standing dispute between Anna Freud and Melanie Klein, both pioneers in child analysis, was threatening to split the British Psycho-Analytic Society, and came to a head during World War II. There were several psychoanalytic factions in London; one was made up of Anna Freud's supporters and one of Melanie Klein's, and there was an "independent group," in which Bowlby became very active. Indeed, he played a leading role in preventing the society from splitting. Throughout his life he took a very critical view of ideological or dogmatic schools of thought and considered involvement in democratic processes to be important.

During World War II, Bowlby worked with a group of army psychoanalysts and psychiatrists whose primary responsibility was the psychological testing of young officers. He was also able to write an influential paper that dealt with environmental influences on early childhood development and was based on his prewar experience with young thieves at the Child Guidance Clinic. He studied 44 cases in all, evaluated notes and records, and published his findings in the article "Forty-

Four Juvenile Thieves: Their Characters and Home Life" (1944; reprint, 1946). In this work he sought to clarify how early emotional trauma resulting from the experience of loss and separation could affect the development of disturbed behavior. Even then, Bowlby was convinced that children's actual early experiences in the relationship to their mother could play a fundamental role in development, and that neither the Oedipus complex and its resolution nor sexuality was solely responsible for a child's emotional development.

Shortly after the war ended, Bowlby was asked to set up a department for child psychotherapy at the Tavistock Clinic. His enormous organizational talents came to the fore both at the Tavistock and within the British Psycho-Analytic Society, as did his ability to find financial means for a variety of purposes, including research.

James Robertson and Mary Ainsworth, among others, joined Bowlby's new research team. Both would prove to be of lasting importance as colleagues and in the subsequent development of attachment theory. Robertson had worked under Anna Freud as a "boilerman" at her residential nursery, and had been introduced there to techniques for observing children. Later he studied psychiatric social work, and eventually received psychoanalytic training under Anna Freud herself. He quickly became conversant with Bowlby's idea that actual early environmental influences were of crucial importance in the development of children.

During his collaboration with Bowlby, Robertson became distressed at having to observe hospitalized children without being able to intervene. He therefore decided to produce a technically very simple but very moving and impressive documentary film, titled *A Two Year Old Goes to Hospital* (Bowlby, Robertson, & Rosenbluth, 1952; Robertson, 1952). Bowlby made sure the film was scientifically impeccable. This film follows the behavioral changes (protest, despair, and detachment) in a 2-year-old girl admitted to the hospital without her mother. At that time, the phases of children's reactions to separation from their mothers, already identified by Robertson and Bowlby, were not generally known, but were demonstrated for all to see in the film. The film's reception was very mixed. Melanie Klein's proponents, for example, ascribed the reactions of the 2-year-old in the film to her unconscious fantasies about her mother and not to the separation itself. However, Bowlby and Robertson used this film to change visiting practices in children's hospitals, first in London and then in many other countries around the world. Today, while it is not yet a universal standard to admit mothers to pediatric hospitals where their small children are inpatients, this is now seen as an important goal and is no longer questioned on theoretical grounds.[1]

Another major collaborator was the Canadian Mary Ainsworth. She had received her degree in Toronto and was already an assistant professor when she came to London with her husband. In her doctoral dissertation she had examined Blatz's (1940) "security theory," according to which full emotional development requires that each human being be able to develop a fundamental trust in an important reference figure. Ainsworth joined Bowlby's research group in London with these insights and was inspired both by his thinking and by Robertson's observational techniques.

In 1949, during the period of turbulent dispute over his new theses, Bowlby was asked by the World Health Organization (WHO) to write a report on the condition of the many children left homeless and orphaned after the war (Bowlby, 1951, 1953, 1973). He used this opportunity not only to review field research on the emotional condition of war orphans but also to make contact with American developmental psychologists, since he was not trained in that field. The knowledge he gained from his involvement in the WHO report encouraged him in his theory building. It was this report that gave him the idea to look for alternative explanations of attachment and led to his interest in ethology.

After becoming familiar with the work of Lorenz (1943) and Tinbergen (1952), Bowlby in his reflections on attachment was increasingly influenced by ethological research. He found his own observations confirmed in Lorenz's (1935/1951) field studies of imprinting and later in Harlow's (1958) work on the effects of maternal separation and deprivation on the social behavior of infant rhesus macaques.

Bowlby eventually presented his thoughts about attachment for public discussion in a series of three lectures before the British Psycho-Analytic Society (published in Bowlby, 1958, 1960a, 1960b). In his groundbreaking article "The Nature of the Child's Tie to His Mother,"

Bowlby (1958) laid out for the first time his conviction that there is a biologically based system of attachment that is responsible for the powerful emotional relationship between mother and child. Reactions to his ideas ranged from extraordinarily skeptical to openly dismissive. The sharpest criticism of his theory was that his concepts abandoned the metatheory of psychoanalysis, namely, drive theory. Bowlby had counterposed a new set of ideas to traditional drive theory, which held that the oral satisfactions of nursing are primarily responsible for the development of a child's attachment to the mother. At that time it was completely unthinkable, according to psychoanalytic theory, that there might be an independent biologically anchored motivational basis for the development of attachment that did not derive either from conflict or from sexuality (A. Freud, 1960; Schur, 1960; Spitz, 1960). Distressed by the direction Bowlby's ideas were taking, Anna Freud wrote to a colleague: "Dr. Bowlby is too valuable a person to get lost to psychoanalysis." Klein's proponents also greeted Bowlby's concepts with suspicion.

Following the publication of Bowlby's seminal attachment papers, his relationship with Ainsworth and their joint scientific activities became fundamentally important in the further development of attachment theory. Although initially skeptical of the ethological foundations of attachment theory, Ainsworth had realized their appropriateness while undertaking a short-term longitudinal study of infants and mothers in Uganda, where she had accompanied her husband in 1954. In Uganda she was able to conduct the kind of field study that she had already decided to do while collaborating with Robertson in London. Ainsworth's observational techniques, though compatible with ethology, thus actually stemmed from Robertson and indirectly from Anna Freud (Bretherton, 1992). Ainsworth observed the relationship between small children and their mothers during 2-hour visits in their homes every 2 weeks accompanied by an interpreter (Ainsworth, 1967), making very detailed records both of the mother's care-giving behavior and the child's attachment and separation behavior.

After her return from Uganda, and as Professor of Developmental Psychology at the Johns Hopkins University, Ainsworth conducted a longitudinal study of infants in Baltimore. Again, during monthly home visits, she and her collaborators observed the mother's caregiving and infants' interactive behavior in minute detail and in highly varied every-day situations. Ainsworth eventually developed a test-like standard procedure, which she called the "Strange Situation," to study children's attachment and separation behavior in a laboratory setting (Ainsworth & Wittig, 1969). At the same time, Bowlby published the first volume of his trilogy, *Attachment and Loss*, titled *Attachment* (1969), incorporating Ainsworth's as yet unpublished results. Over the next several years, Bowlby wrote a second theoretical volume, titled *Separation, Anxiety and Anger* (1973), in which he described the effects of the experience of separation, and then a third volume on the importance of loss, titled *Loss, Sadness and Depression* (1980). This trilogy comprises the theoretical foundation of attachment theory.

Further empirical support for the theory came from numerous longitudinal studies by developmental psychologists. By then, Ainsworth had a host of doctoral students, a whole new generation of attachment researchers, including among others Silvia Bell, Mary Main, Robert Marvin, Mary Blehar, Inge Bretherton, and Everett Waters (an undergraduate, who helped as research assistant). When Everett Waters went to the University of Minnesota as a graduate student he acquainted Alan Sroufe with the Strange Situation (Bretherton, 1992). This led to an influential and still ongoing longitudinal study. Klaus and Karin Grossmann from Germany visited after having heard about Ainsworth, both to study the Strange Situation and to learn more about attachment research. The two still ongoing longitudinal attachment studies that they subsequently undertook in Germany laid a significant foundation for subsequent European research into attachment.

Later, a special semistructured interview was designed to study adults. This "Adult Attachment Interview" (AAI) was developed by Carol George (see George, Kaplan, & Main, 1985) in conjunction with her doctoral dissertation. She did not find anything of interest by analyzing specific answers given to the separate interview questions, but Main and Goldwyn (1985) discovered that *how* mothers processed and discussed their childhood experiences was related to their infants' behavior in the Strange Situation. This made it possible to ask adults about their early attachment experiences and, through a close analysis of the transcribed interview text, to draw conclusions about their attitudes toward attachment. In addition to examining the development of early childhood attachment by observing behavior, researchers were now able to move to the representational level, by examining how attachment experiences were recalled by adults (Main, Kaplan, & Cassidy, 1985).

Various attempts were also made to examine 3- to 6-year-old children's attachment-related representational world. Kaplan (1987) and Slough and Greenberg (1991) used a revision of Klagsbrun and Bowlby's (1976) Separation Anxiety Test (SAT), adapted from Hansburg's version for adolescents (1972). During this test, young children are presented with a set of pictures that portray situations of separation and loss, and the coherence and emotional openness of children's verbal responses are analyzed. Other researchers developed short incomplete stories focusing on attachment issues that were acted out with small family figures (Bretherton, Ridgeway, & Cassidy, 1990; Cassidy, 1988). Children's narrative and play responses were analyzed using a procedure similar to that adopted for the SAT by Kaplan (1987; see Main, Kaplan, & Cassidy, 1985). The story completion method was further elaborated by Bretherton, in collaboration with Oppenheim, Buchsbaum, and Emde, as the MacArthur Story Stem Battery (MSSB; Bretherton, Oppenheim, Buchsbaum, & Emde, 1990). Although the assessment of attachment at the representational level was not the sole purpose of the MSSB, Oppenheim and colleagues correlated it with other behavioral measures (Emde, Oppenheim, Nir, & Warren, 1997; Oppenheim, Emde, & Warren, 1997).

A complete overview of the current state of empirical attachment research is hardly possible. However, significant work on the various constructs of attachment research, which will be described in the next chapter, has been summarized by a Dutch research group under van IJzendoorn (e.g., 1995a). Extensive reviews can be found in the *Handbook of Attachment*, edited by Cassidy and Shaver (1999).

In Bowlby's conception, the quality of attachment as it develops during the first months of life between an infant and the primary attachment figure is not something fixed but can change dramatically over the life cycle as a result of emotional experiences in new relationships. Seen in this light, attachment is an emotional bond that develops during childhood but whose influence is not limited to this early developmental phase, but rather embraces all further stages of life. As such, attachment represents an emotional base that extends into old age (Parkes et al., 1991). Attachment theory has also affected our understanding of the importance of death and dying. In her work, Kübler-Ross (1974) occasionally made use of its theoretical and therapeutic approaches.

During the last years of his life, Bowlby once again turned his attention to the therapeutic application of his theory (Bowlby, 1988). He felt it particularly important to prevent the development of psychopathological patterns of attachment in the early adult–child relationship, as well as in psychotherapeutic work generally.

As a result of empirical (especially prospective longitudinal) studies, attachment theory is today one of the most solidly founded theories of human development. Even though it does not examine all areas equally (and may, at least in the early years, have neglected some aspects of sexuality, aggression, and the importance of the father), it has nonetheless served as a considerable building block and has contributed to the understanding of human development throughout the life cycle.

~

## THE DEVELOPMENT OF THE CONCEPTS OF ATTACHMENT THEORY[2]

### Basic Assumptions of Attachment Theory

*The Definition of Attachment and Attachment Theory*

Bowlby viewed mother and infant as participants in a self-regulating and mutually interacting system. As conceived by him, the attachment system was a regulatory system within the child interacting with the complementary caregiving system within the parent. The attachment relationship between mother and child differs from the parent–child relationship as a whole in that "attachment" is understood to be one part of the complex system of the relationship that includes other aspects such as teaching and play.[3]

Attachment theory combines contributions from ethology, developmental psychology, systems theory, and psychoanalysis. It focuses on the fundamental early influences on the emotional development of the child and attempts to explain the development of and changes in strong emotional attachments between individuals throughout the life cycle.

## The Attachment System

According to Bowlby, the attachment system represents a very basic and genetically anchored motivational and behavioral system that is in some way biologically preformed, that serves a survival function for the child, and that is activated after birth in relation to specific attachment figures.

The infant and young child seeks closeness, especially to his mother, when he experiences anxiety. This may occur when, for example, he is separated from his mother, encounters threatening unfamiliar situations or strange persons, experiences physical pain, or feels overwhelmed by his fantasies, as in nightmares. The infant or young child hopes to find safety, protection, and security in proximity to his mother. This search for closeness may be accomplished by visual contact with the mother or, especially, by seeking close bodily contact with her. The child is always an active partner in the interaction, signaling when the needs for closeness and protection are present and must be satisfied.

## Sensitivity and Attachment Quality

"Sensitive behavior" by an attachment figure requires the ability to attune to the child's signals (e.g., crying), interpret them correctly (e.g., as proximity- and contact-seeking), and satisfy them promptly and appropriately. Ideally this "sensitive behavior" occurs countless times in the interactions of daily life (see also the discussion of "The Concept of Sensitivity" later in this section).[4] An infant is likely to develop a secure attachment to an attachment figure whose sensitive caregiving behavior satisfies his needs in the manner described above. On the other hand, if these needs are not met in his interaction with the attachment figure, or if they are met only partially or inconsistently—for example, in an unpredictable manner that fluctuates between interference in the form of overreaction, overalertness, or overstimulation and extremely frustrating denial by rejection and ignoring—insecure attachment is more apt to develop.

### The Hierarchy of Attachment Figures

If the principal attachment figure is absent during a threatening situation, or if the child is separated from her, he will react with sadness, crying, and anger, and actively attempt to seek her out. During his first year of life, the infant forms an attachment to a hierarchy of figures who will be sought in a particular order according to their availability and the level of separation anxiety that is experienced. For example, if the mother, as principal attachment figure, is not available in times of danger, the child may then fall back on a secondary attachment figure (such as the father) for emotional security. The greater the pain or anxiety—in case of serious accident or illness, for example—the more insistently and uncompromisingly the child will insist on the presence of the primary attachment figure and not allow himself to be comforted by secondary ones.

### Internal Working Models

During the first year of life, out of the many interactional experiences and transactions between mother and infant that involve experiences of separation and re-establishment of closeness, the infant develops representational models of his interactions with his mother and of corresponding affects that Bowlby termed "internal working models"[5] (Bowlby, 1969; Bretherton & Munholland, 1999; Main, Kaplan, & Cassidy, 1985). These models make the interaction of attachment figure and child in attachment situations predictable. During the first year the child learns that, when he is in danger, if he cries and seeks out his attachment figure as his "safe haven," she will be there (or not there) for him and answer his need for attachment with a certain characteristic closeness or distance and a comprehensive repertoire of behaviors. Separate working models are developed for each individual attachment figure—father and mother, for example.

In the beginning such working models are flexible, but over the further course of development they become increasingly stable. It is believed that on the basis of these relationship models, which have both conscious and unconscious aspects, individuals develop one preferred attachment strategy of relating (Main, 1995). It is still an unsolved problem in attachment theory how different working models of mother and father contribute to the development of one preferred strategy. It is easy to understand, however, how a secure and stable attachment representation would become part of an individual's psychic structure and thereby contribute to psychic stability.

### The Stability of Attachment Representations

I assume that over the course of a person's life a stable (secure or insecure) attachment strategy may become more or less distilled as a "leading representation," either as a result of important attachments to other persons or because of dire experiences such as loss or other trauma. Main (1995) believes, on the basis of findings obtained with the AAI, that most adults develop a specific strategy for processing attachment-related thoughts and feelings, also termed a "state of mind" with respect to attachment. By this she appears to mean a regulatory system that wards off (dismisses) attachment thoughts, feelings, and behaviors or exaggerates them (preoccupation). However, change in this regulatory strategy becomes increasingly difficult with advancing age. Hence, we find that adolescents' responses to the AAI are predictable from their attachment quality to mother at the age of 12 months, but we also see discontinuities in attachment quality over the lifespan (see also Zimmermann, Spangler, Schicche, & Becker-Stoll, 1995). Moreover, irrespective of attachment quality, we can assume that the internal working models of an adolescent are much more sophisticated than those of a 1-year-old.

### The Exploratory System

The need for attachment stands in seeming opposition to the infant's need to explore, which Bowlby (1969) viewed as another important behavioral system.[6] Although the attachment system and the exploratory system originate in opposing motivations, they exist in a state of interdependence.

According to Bowlby, an infant can explore his environment adequately and move away from his mother without distress if she permits him to do so in her role as his secure emotional base. In Bowlby's view, the child therefore does not need to become distressed if the mother is available and responsive. Secure attachment is a precondition of an infant's ability to explore his environment and experience himself as an agent and self-effective individual.[7]

From the very beginning, and increasingly as the child's motor development progresses (from the crawling stage at 7–8 months onward), the mother must make room for the infant's wish to explore while, in my view, simultaneously setting limits on it.[8] At the same time, the mother must be consistently accessible as a secure base so that the infant may gain reassurance from her while exploring; this has been described by Emde and Sorce (1983) as "social referencing." When the infant returns to his mother from his explorations, he must feel emotionally accepted by her. Mahler metaphorically called this behavior "emotional refueling" (Mahler, Pine, & Bergman, 1975).

### The Interplay between the Attachment System and the Exploratory System

Once the child's attachment needs are satisfied and he is able to experience emotional security with an attachment figure, the attachment system is assuaged, and the infant can indulge his curiosity in the form of exploratory behavior. In so doing, he is able to tolerate greater or lesser degrees of distance from his attachment figure without experiencing emotional distress.[9] If the attachment system is activated either because the distance becomes too great or because of fear-provoking discoveries, exploration will become increasingly limited, and the child will seek spatial or even physical closeness to the attachment figure, who represents his most secure emotional base. A sensitive attachment figure accepts the infant's regulation of distance and closeness and can feel confident that her child will seek proximity to her in situations of stress. If this expected behavior does not occur, it has presumably been actively suppressed as a result of experienced rejection. Once the child feels adequately reassured, exploratory activity is activated and does not have to be forced. Initiation and control of attachment and exploration behavior emanate from the child himself.

If a mother clings to her infant, she may indeed create a close relationship—but not a secure attachment. By not giving her infant sufficient scope to exercise his need to explore, she may thereby frustrate him. This can occur out of fear that the child might injure himself in his exploration or out of her own fear of being abandoned.

### Goal-Corrected Partnership

By preschool age, a so-called goal-corrected partnership develops between a child and an attachment figure. Through bargaining and negotiating about his attachment-related goals the child can now maintain a balance between the need for attachment and the desire to explore. Ideally, the balance between attachment and exploration exists in infancy, but because of increasing social-cognitive and verbal sophistication, preschool children can better negotiate their needs for closeness and security than infants, because they can now take the mother's goals into account to some extent. The sensitive mother is goal-corrected from the beginning, but the relationship becomes a goal-corrected partnership only when the child is also able to pay attention to maternal goals and not only to his own (Bowlby, 1969). In such a relationship both partners communicate the goals that are emotionally important to them, attend to their partner's interests (which may conflict with their own), reflect, and then finally negotiate and adjust common goals in partnership.[10]

### Attachment and Exploration throughout the Life Cycle

The reciprocal relationship between attachment and exploration is, according to attachment theory, a phenomenon that endures well beyond infancy. Bowlby saw it as a lifelong process. The tension between the two poles of attachment and exploration must constantly be balanced like a seesaw, because attachment and exploration relate to each other as thesis to antithesis.

*Transgenerational Transmission of Attachment Patterns*

The infant's attachment quality depends upon the "state of mind" or attachment strategy of the attachment figures who care for and play with him. There is a connection between the quality of the attachment representations in the parental generation and the attachment quality that develops in infancy (Fonagy, Steele, & Steele, 1991; Main et al., 1985; Steele & Steele, 1994).

*Secure Attachment as a Protective Factor*

Secure attachment developed during infancy is thought to have a protective function. Longitudinal studies have shown that it promotes prosocial behavior and the development of a psychic resilience that can withstand a certain level of stress (Main & Weston, 1981).

## The Concept of Sensitivity

In this section I will explain the concept of sensitivity and other important concepts of attachment theory in greater detail. According to attachment theory, the sensitivity of the caregiver is an important foundation for the quality of attachment developed by an infant in the first year of life.

The concept of sensitivity was primarily developed by Mary Ainsworth (see Ainsworth, Bell, & Stayton, 1974). She had first formulated the concept of maternal sensitivity while interviewing mothers in Uganda, and further elaborated it during her subsequent study in Baltimore with a small group of 26 infants. These infants were observed with their mothers and other family members at home across the first year of life. At the end of the first year, that is, after one year of home visits lasting several hours each, Ainsworth carried out a standardized protocol that she had developed for assessing separation behavior in the laboratory, the so-called Strange Situation. She found that children of mothers who had exhibited sensitive caregiving behavior at home demonstrated particular behavior patterns in the Strange Situation. These were later called "secure" because of their correlations with interaction patterns shown during home observations. The opposite finding—more frequent insecure attachment—occurred in children of less sensitive mothers (Ainsworth, Blehar, Waters, & Wall, 1978).

Ainsworth and colleagues (1974) characterized sensitive caregiving behavior as follows:

1. The mother must be able to attune to her infant's signals with attentiveness. Hesitation in her ability to attune may result from external or internal preoccupation with her own needs and well-being.
2. She must appropriately interpret the signals from the perspective of the infant. For example, she must decipher the meaning of the child's crying (from hunger, illness, pain, boredom). There is a danger that the infant's signals may be distorted or incorrectly interpreted as a result of her own needs, or by projection of these needs onto the child.
3. She must respond appropriately to the signals. For example, she must ascertain the correct amount of nourishment, soothe the child, if possible, or offer play stimuli without burdening the mother–child interaction either by overstimulation or understimulation.
4. Her reaction must be prompt, taking place within a time period that does not cause intolerable frustration for the child. The time period during which an infant can wait to be nursed is very short during the first weeks of life but becomes longer over the course of the first year.

In my clinical experience, it is relatively easy for many attachment figures and caregivers to perceive an infant's signals more or less sensitively, although Ainsworth had mothers in her sample who found this difficult. Crying may be easier to detect than some other signals. Nevertheless, during home visits as well as in clinical observations of the mother–child interaction, the amount of time that passes before the mother registers the child's signals (crying, wailing, complaining) can be observed to vary in length.[11] Particularly brief or muted signals from the child will only be perceptible to very sensitive mothers.[12] Interpreting these signals correctly is much more difficult than it is to realize that an infant is crying. I know from the seminars we conducted for parents in Ulm (Germany) that many parents initially have a difficult time interpreting crying, particularly with their first child. Most mothers learned fairly quickly to differentiate among the kinds of crying that stemmed from hunger, boredom, protest, pain, a dirty diaper, or overstimulation, but needed a trial-and-error period before being able to correctly connect the signal of crying to the desires and motivations underlying it (Papoušek, 1994).

Most attachment figures must also learn the appropriate response to the correctly interpreted signal. With each of their children, they must ascertain at what point a particular child's need for food, physical contact, stimulation, or sleep is adequately satisfied. Experiences with the first child cannot simply be generalized to later siblings, because every child is temperamentally different, copes with irritation differently, and makes wishes and needs known in different ways (Crockenberg, 1986).

In our German experience, most parents, even today, fear that they may spoil their children during the first year. In their worst-case fantasies, they see their child as a "spoiled monster" or a "little tyrant," to whose every wish they will have to cater. For this reason, many parents do not necessarily see a quick reaction to their child's wishes and signals as desirable, although their general capacities for sensitive behavior can be seen in the clinical examination of mother–child and father–child interaction. They are convinced that the child must learn as early as possible to endure frustration.

Parents' and experts' opinions differ widely about what levels of frustration promote optimal growth and what constitutes an excessive demand on the child's ability to regulate his own affect. Over the course of the first year of life, infants become increasingly able to defer gratification of their needs. Here, too, parental sensitivity is required with increasing demands placed on the infant's ability to wait, thereby frustrating the child to the point where his ability to regulate himself is exhausted. For this reason, the basic requirements for the prompt satisfaction of needs must be continually redefined at each age level. That is what Ainsworth's sensitive mothers were able to do; hence, their relationships with their infants were more harmonious in the final quarter of the first year of life.

Sensitivity differs from spoiling or overprotectiveness in that sensitive parents support their child in his increasing autonomy and growing ability to communicate. Infants of sensitive mothers, examined during their first year of life, were able to play and explore their surroundings more on their own, but they also more readily sought comfort and security from their mothers when afraid or stressed. Their interactions with their mothers were characterized by less anxiety and irritation. They were consistently able to separate from their mothers after allowing her to comfort them for a short period of time, and they were more prepared to cooperate with the limits their mothers set (Ainsworth et al., 1978; Grossmann, Grossmann, Spangler, Suess, & Unzner, 1985; van IJzendoorn & Hubbard, 2000).

Infants of less sensitive mothers either did not ask for their mother's support, or showed such marked signs of anxiety, irritation, or aggression that they were hardly able to play at a distance from their mothers, nor could they be soothed by her or engage in play in her presence. They were also less likely to accept the limitations placed on them by their mother (Grossmann et al., 1985; Stayton, Hogan, & Ainsworth, 1973).

### Sensitivity Training for Parents-to-Be

With Ainsworth's call for sensitive caregiving behavior in mind, my colleague Anna Buchheim and I set up a sensitivity training workshop for expectant parents in Ulm. Couples expecting their first child were told about the results of infant research during five evening sessions at our Institute for Early Childhood Development and Parent–Child Research (a building we called the "Yellow House").[13] One of our focal points was Ainsworth's concept of sensitivity. The idea was that the parents should learn to evaluate parental caregiving behavior by watching videotaped examples and thereby become more sensitized to what constitutes sensitive parental care. Three, 6, and 12 weeks after the infant's birth, we made separate videotapes of the mother and father engaged in diapering and play. Afterwards, we watched the "diapering videos" during the sensitivity training session, and analyzed them sequence by sequence with each parent individually. The goal was to enable the parents to attune

accurately to their child's signals and to see and interpret their own behavior, thereby helping them to learn how to interact more sensitively
with their child. Reinforcement and respect for the parents, as well as
tact and a validating attitude, were fundamental to the training whenever insensitive sequences of interaction were found and analyzed.
When viewing scenes in which parents showed less sensitivity, we all
considered how they might interpret their own behavior as well as their
child's actions and reactions. Particularly when the projection of their
own wishes and feelings had a negative effect on interaction with the
child, we supported them in finding alternative explanations for their
child's behavior.

Evaluation of the results allowed us to conclude that the parents in
the study group perceived their children's signals more sensitively and,
above all, viewed their own behavior more critically than did parents in
a control group that did not receive sensitivity training. The parents in
the control group, whom we had invited only to make a diapering-
playing video when their child was 3 months old, more often idealized
their own behavior and overestimated their sensitivity to the child's
signals.

Intervention studies similarly designed to improve parental sensitivity have been carried out in the United States and The Netherlands.
These indicate that maternal sensitivity can be positively influenced by
focused interventions both in the home and in sensitivity training
sessions with the videotapes (Bakermans-Kranenburg, Juffer, & van
IJzendoorn, 1998; Egeland & Erickson, 1993; Erickson, 2000; van den
Boom, 1990, 1994).

## The Concept of Attachment Quality in Children

The quality of child attachment is often studied by carrying out the
Strange Situation protocol. This standardized protocol has been used
around the world in highly varied social settings and has been shown to
be a valid and reliable instrument. The mother, her child, and a strange
person participate in the Strange Situation, a defined sequence of episodes during the course of which mother and child are twice separated
and then reunited after several minutes. In the process, the child's
attachment system is activated, and the quality of attachment can be re-

liably evaluated through observation of the behavior between mother and child (Ainsworth et al., 1978).

Although the Strange Situation can be criticized on the grounds that it captures only one specific aspect of mother–child interaction—that it constitutes a "snapshot"—and that its evaluation is specifically geared to the behavior of the child while ignoring maternal reactions, it has been shown to be valid and to predict theoretically important outcomes (for a review, see Weinfeld, Sroufe, Egeland, & Carlson, 1999; for a critique, see Fox, Kimmerly, & Schafer, 1991).

The Strange Situation is conducted when the child is between 12 and 18 months of age, in a playroom specially outfitted for the purpose. Neither the mother nor the child is familiar with the setting, so it represents a "strange situation" for both. The entire procedure consists of eight episodes, each of which lasts for 3 minutes and is videotaped for subsequent evaluation (Ainsworth & Wittig, 1969; Ainsworth et al., 1978).

- *First and second episode*: Mother and child enter the unfamiliar playroom. After a short period of acclimation, the curious child begins to explore the unfamiliar and attractive toys. The mother assists her child in playing only to the extent that it's absolutely necessary. In general, the mother sits in a chair and can observe her child playing. Some mothers read while their child is playing at their feet.

- *Third episode*: A stranger enters the room, and does not speak at first. After 1 minute the person begins to talk to the mother, and a brief dialogue ensues. The children generally react to the stranger with curiosity or slight anxiety and decrease their distance from their mother; or they may become somewhat more inhibited in their play. During the third minute of this episode, the stranger tries to make contact with the child by offering to play with him or her (the stranger is lively and animated during this last minute of the episode, though not coercive).

- *Fourth episode*: When she hears a tapping signal, the mother leaves the room without saying goodbye to the child, as instructed. We generally observe that the child follows his mother with his eyes, calls after her, or even begins to cry. Sometimes the child follows the mother to the door, behind which she disappears for a short time. The stranger tries to console the child or to divert him with play. This effort succeeds to varying degrees, and sometimes not at all. The episode is curtailed if the child cannot be comforted.

• *Fifth episode*: After a 3-minute separation, the mother calls the child's name and then comes back into the room. She picks him up and tries to console him as needed. As soon as the child has quieted down, she allows him to begin playing again. In general children themselves want to return to playing. The stranger leaves the room shortly after the mother returns.

• *Sixth episode*: A second separation occurs after 3 minutes. After saying "Bye-bye, I'll be back," the mother again leaves the room when she hears the tapping signal, and the child is left completely alone. Frequently, we now observe a stronger separation reaction in the child, whose attachment system has already been activated by the first separation. The child often follows the mother, calls out for her, begins to cry, and shows other signs of emotional distress.

• *Seventh episode*: After the 3 minutes of separation (or earlier if the child is very distressed) the stranger again enters the room, instead of the mother, whom the child expects. The stranger makes another attempt to console or divert the child.

• *Eighth episode*: The mother returns after a further 3 minutes, or earlier if the child is inconsolable. If he cries or approaches her, she soothes the child by taking him into her arms. Many, but not all, children return to play after a relatively short period of consolation, usually about 3 minutes.

When 1-year-old children were first observed in the Strange Situation, Ainsworth and her colleagues noted various reactions and behaviors that could reliably be classified into three types of attachment quality (1978; Ainsworth, 1985). In subsequent studies by other researchers using the Strange Situation a fourth classification was described.

## The Classification of Infant Attachment Quality

### "Secure" Attachment

These children display clear attachment behavior after both the first and the second separation from the mother. They call after her, follow her, look for her—sometimes persistently—and many finally start to cry, showing clear signs of distress. They react with happiness when the mother returns, reach out with their arms, want to be consoled, and seek physical contact. Shortly thereafter they become calm and are able to return to play.

### "Avoidant" Attachment

These children react to separation with little protest and display no clear attachment behavior, such as following the mother to the door or crying. In general, they continue to play, although perhaps with less curiosity or persistence. Occasionally they follow the mother with their eyes when she leaves the room, so it is clear that they do register her disappearance. After her return, they are apt to react to her with avoidance, and they do not ask to be taken into her arms. Usually there is no intense physical contact.

### "Ambivalent" Attachment

These children demonstrate the greatest distress after separation and cry intensely. Their mothers upon return are not able to calm them quickly. It generally takes these children longer to achieve emotional equilibrium. Sometimes they are not able to return to play, even after several minutes. When their mothers pick them up, the children express a desire for physical contact and closeness while at the same time behaving aggressively toward their mothers (kicking, hitting, pushing, or turning away).

### Disorganized Behavior Pattern (Additional Classification)

After Ainsworth and colleagues (1978) had identified the secure, avoidant, and ambivalent attachment classifications in the Strange Situation, a number of children in other studies could not be placed into any of these three categories. Typical peculiarities of behavior were later identified in these children, who were described as "insecure–disorganized/disoriented" by Main and Solomon (1990). Even infants classified as securely attached on the basis of their main behavioral strategy may

demonstrate short periods of disorganized behavior, such as running toward the mother, stopping short halfway, and then turning around and
running away from her, increasing their distance. That is, the movements of such children may appear to "freeze." In addition, Main and
Solomon observed repetitive stereotyped behavior and movement patterns. They interpreted these behaviors as a sign that the child's attachment system had been activated but could not express itself in clear behavioral strategies.

This "disorganized/disoriented" category may be assigned to a
child as an additional code to the three attachment patterns termed
secure, insecure–avoidant and insecure–ambivalent. As physiological
measurements indicate, children demonstrating a disorganized pattern
in the Strange Situation experience high stress, similar to that found in
insecurely attached avoidant and ambivalent children (Spangler &
Grossmann, 1993). This pattern is therefore grouped with the insecure
category if the specific behaviors described above are present to a high
degree.

The disorganized pattern has been found more often than statistically expected in children from clinical high-risk groups, and also in
children whose parents had experienced such traumas as loss, separation, maltreatment, and abuse and had carried these experiences into
their relationship with the child (Main & Hesse, 1990).

The behaviors described as "disorganized" are also reminiscent of
reactions seen in infants and small children in at-risk samples, such as
premature children (Minde, 1993b) or victims of early childhood abuse
(Carlson, Cicchetti, Barnett, & Braunwald, 1989) and deprivation
(Lyons-Ruth, Alpern, & Repacholi, 1993; Lyons-Ruth, Repacholi, McLeod,
& Silva, 1991). It may be assumed that the differences in disorganized
behavior between nonclinical and clinical samples indicate risk of psychopathology.

The overall distribution of infant attachment patterns across 21
studies with nonclinical groups in the United States has been as follows:
67% of infants were classified as secure, 21% as insecure–avoidant, and
12% as insecure–ambivalent; corresponding percentages for western
Europe, based on nine nonclinical samples, are 66% secure, 28% avoidant, and 6% ambivalent (van IJzendoorn & Sagi, 1999). As already

noted, the percentage of children demonstrating disorganized behavior is greater in clinical samples. The greater the infant's risk level (including biological risk), or the greater the parents' risk level (e.g., psychological risk) that manifests in their interaction with their children, the more distinctly or frequently will disorganized behavior be found across all attachment categories (Grossmann, 1988).

## Correlations of Strange Situation Behavior with Other Variables

A moderately strong correlation was found in several studies between sensitive caregiving behavior by the attachment figure and attachment security found in the children at 1 year of age. Sensitive mothers more frequently have infants that show the secure pattern in the Strange Situation, and less sensitive mothers more frequently have infants showing the insecure patterns (van IJzendoorn, Juffer, & Duyvesteyn, 1995). Whereas Ainsworth and colleagues (1978) reported highly significant correlations between the sensitivity of a mother's care and the attachment quality of children in the pioneering Baltimore study, this finding has been weaker in subsequent studies. The current state of research assumes that only 12% of the variance in children's attachment patterns is explained by maternal sensitivity (see meta-analysis by De Wolff & van IJzendoorn, 1997), but this result must be viewed with caution. In the studies included in this meta-analysis, the instruments and situations used to measure sensitivity varied widely and were not necessarily based on Ainsworth's definition. That is, an important condition for meta-analysis—the comparability of studies—might not have been fulfilled.

Moreover, in considering these correlations, the genetic disposition of the infant's regulatory systems may be a contributory factor in the formation of attachment quality, and should be viewed as the infant's contribution to the interaction. Children characterized by higher irritability in early infancy and weaker orientation reactions in the first few weeks after birth were more frequently evaluated as insecurely attached in the Strange Situation, even though their mothers' behavior was of average sensitivity (Grossmann et al., 1985).

As soon as the influence of infantile characteristics on attachment pattern had been understood, a critical discussion ensued about whether or not differences in the attachment behavior of particular children could be adequately explained by differences in temperament (Fox, 1992; Fox et al., 1991; Sroufe, 1985; Vaughn & Bost, 1999). Today it is assumed that temperament, or the child's genetically based predispositions and behavioral characteristics, contribute to the mother–child interaction both during the first year and in the Strange Situation (van IJzendoorn & Bakermans-Kranenburg, 1997), but may be counteracted by maternal sensitivity. An agitated or uncontrollably crying infant, or one with marked eating or sleep problems, for instance, may put a strain on even the average sensitive mother's behavior, and possibly overtax her. As a clinician I have observed how quickly the mother–child interaction can go awry with such infants, and how major secondary behavioral difficulties can result (Papoušek, 1996).

Psychophysiological tests have shown that all infants react to some degree with physiological stress—such as elevation of the heart rate—to separation from their mothers in the Strange Situation. The children classified as insecure–avoidant, who appeared so calm from the outside, and to whom extraordinary adaptability, greater independence, and a more placid temperament were initially ascribed, were shown to exhibit even higher saliva cortisol levels, a measurement of the experience of stress, than either the securely attached children or those thought to be insecurely-ambivalently attached. For this reason, the insecure–avoidant behavior pattern must be understood as a defensive or adaptive achievement, the consequence of which is an elevated psychophysiological, hormonal, and immunological stress test reaction (Reite & Field, 1985; Schieche & Spangler, 1994; Spangler, 1998; Spangler & Grossmann, 1993; Spangler & Schieche, 1995).

## The Concept of Attachment Representation

After the Strange Situation, as a method for assessing the attachment quality of infants and small children had become well established and validated, George and colleagues developed a semistructured interview, now called the "Adult Attachment Interview" (AAI), to capture the childhood attachment experiences of adults (George, Kaplan, & Main, 1985; see Hesse, 1999). The purpose was to explore whether the parents' childhood experiences of attachment contributed to their children's attachment quality. In this interview, adults are asked about their childhood, their relationships with parents, and particularly their memories of concrete situations in which their parents responded to their distress and comforted them. Parents are also asked about the significance of separations and losses, and to evaluate the influence *their* parents had on their personality development. Further questions focus on changes in the relationship to their parents over time as well as the ways in which they currently deal with separations from their own actual or imagined children (the Appendix, reprinted from Hesse, 1999, provides a brief précis of the AAI protocol).

On the basis of an evaluation method developed by Main and Goldwyn, adult attachment interviews can be classified into four categories: secure or free–autonomous, dismissing, preoccupied, and unresolved (Main & Goldwyn, 1984; for a summary, see Hesse, 1999). In generating this evaluation, Main and Goldwyn recognized that responses to the AAI questions are often influenced by defensive processes, leading to moments of incoherence in the narrative that are not registered or corrected by the interviewee (as evident in the examples from Buchheim, Brisch, & Kächele, 1998, that are cited verbatim below). Main, Kaplan, and Cassidy (1985; Main, 1995) discovered that classifications of the parental narratives about attachment in childhood could be predicted from their infants' Strange Situation classifications 5 years earlier.

The AAI evaluations, which require extensive training, are performed by means of an in-depth textual analysis of verbatim transcripts. Their purpose is to assess the organization of an individual's attachment memories and thoughts. Coherence of narrative and of discourse are the primary criteria on which this analysis is based. According to Grice (1975), coherent discourse must meet the criteria of quality (be honest and provide evidence for your statements), of quantity (be brief but complete), of relevance (stay on topic and don't stray from it), and structural comprehensibility (order your ideas and make them understandable).

*Secure (Coherent and Collaborative) Attachment Representation*
*with a Valuing Attitude toward Attachment ("Free Autonomous")*

Securely organized adults generally report positive experiences of attachment with their parents and describe situations in which they experienced loving care and comfort. Even when their childhood experiences were characterized by pain, separation, and losses, they are still able to talk about them in a detailed and thoughtful way, and therefore fulfill Grice's coherence criteria as described above. Additionally, a special evaluative method subsequently developed by Fonagy, Steele, and colleagues (1996) shows that secure AAIs are characterized by a high level of self-reflectiveness.

Main (1995) has suggested that adults who can report negative experiences coherently have gained this ability either from later experiences with an important attachment figure or through psychotherapy. Such people can relive and describe their own painful life events self-reflectively, and in context. It is also possible to document this type of change when comparing a patient's descriptions of childhood experiences given at the beginning of treatment with his or her narratives given at the end of therapy. Main called this kind of secure attachment organization, achieved later in life, "earned secure" (cf. also Pearson, Cohen, Cowan, & Cowan, 1994). It is one of her major insights that a parent's report of adverse childhood experiences per se does not predict his or her infant's Strange Situation classification. What matters is how that adverse childhood is processed and talked about. The verbatim examples below are from Buchheim, Brisch, and Kächele (1998) (I, interviewer; P, participant).

*Example 1 (Based on Positive Childhood Experiences)*

I:  When you were a child, what did you do when you hurt yourself?

P:  Although my mother didn't have much time, something I often had a hard time dealing with, she was always there when I wasn't feeling good.

I:  Can you remember a specific example?

P: I remember, for example, when I hurt my knee; that was during summer vacation. I was about 6 years old, and I went around a curve too fast on my bicycle and was in complete shock. I went right to my mother, who dropped everything she was doing and picked me up and said, "Oh, that must hurt, but it will get better again." You know, when I think about it, I have to say that she did a good job.

### Example of an Avoidant Interview with a Dismissive Attitude toward Attachment ("Dismissing")

These adults characteristically have few memories of their own childhood and ascribe little importance to attachment in their lives. We often find idealizations of relationships to parents, but these idealizations are not confirmed (and sometimes are disconfirmed) by detailed and specific examples.

### Example 2

I: How would you describe your relationship to your parents when you were a child?

P: It was, I was, I had a happy childhood; it was really super.

I: Can you give me an example?

P: It was just a harmonious family, the way you imagine one; just basically so, I mean, just completely normal.

I: What does "normal" mean to you?

P: No idea, I mean, oh dear, well, very warm.

I: Do you have any memories of that?

P: No, I can't remember any; none, no.

I: You can't remember a single concrete example that would describe the warmth?

P: I just remember that it always upset me that I had to wear my sister's hand-me-downs. I remember things like that, but, really, everything was actually super.

## Insecure–Ambivalently Organized Internal Representation ("Entangled or Preoccupied")

The interviewer frequently finds interviews with these adults to be "interminable." The interview is characterized by a plethora of details, entanglements, and contradictory statements. The degree to which the interviewee does not recognize the contradictions in his own statements is remarkable.

*Example 3[14]*

I: How did you perceive your relationship to your mother?

P: Oh, all the stubbornness and self-centeredness, self-will, and also with the narrowness and therefore, I had a very late and very strong conflict. I had to, in order to separate, but she was the one who decided everything for us. Everything in practical matters and at home and so, everything was very clean and "You can't go there," and "I'll do this," and "You will wear that"—she determined that. And "You will play this instrument." Fine, I can understand that, one couldn't do that then, and the school, but, it was very, very advanced, I was so undecided.

I: Can you remember anything else that would describe your relationship back then?

P: And I always want to protect her, and I don't know why. To this day, and, oh well, and actually one has, and I have dreams to this day in which I become absolutely aggressive toward her. This torments me to this day, and . . . and one would still like to, her childhood is so close to me and close enough for me to feel empathetic.

## Insecurely Organized Internal Representation of Attachment with Unresolved Trauma or Loss ("Unresolved")

In the interviews of adults referred for therapy, we have found many statements that are characterized by disorganization and disorientation. Clinicians will recognize such dialogues from their initial conversations with borderline patients, in whom the content of speech, thought processes, and the description of affective experiences tend to break down, and may include manifestly psychotic sequences that can be described as psychic disorganization.

There is evidence in the biographical case histories of such interviewees that they were more likely than others to have experienced trauma such as extreme loss, maltreatment, or abuse, which had not yet been worked through.

*Example 4*

I:  How did you feel about the death of your grandmother at the time?

P:  Oh well, it was pretty bad, I can hardly believe she is dead, I haven't really grasped that she died 2 years ago, and it is as if it was yesterday . . . (*an approximately 30-second pause*) . . .

I:  Did you go to the funeral?

P:  Yes, last year, that was horrible, I don't remember exactly what time of day it was; oh yes, they let the coffin down at exactly 12 o'clock, and Granny had her favorite blouse on, the one with the little red flowers. Her glasses were a little crooked.

I:  You said that the funeral was last year. When did your grandmother die?

P:  Two years ago.

## Attachment across Generations and throughout the Life Cycle

Since Main and colleagues' (1985) discoveries demonstrating correlations between infant attachment classifications and parental AAIs, other attachment researchers have been interested in the question of whether and how attachment quality is transmitted from parents to their children (the transgenerational perspective). They have also been interested in how a particular infant attachment pattern continues to develop over the lifespan (the longitudinal perspective).

Miriam and Howard Steele in London carried out a groundbreaking study that provided important information about the transgenerational transmission of attachment organization (Fonagy et al., 1991; Steele & Steele, 1994). They administered the Adult Attachment Interview to women and their partners during the final 3 months of pregnancy. On the basis of the interview classifications, they were able to reliably predict the quality of the infants' attachment to each parent at 1 year of age. These results have since been replicated in other studies over as many as three generations (Benoit & Parker, 1994; Radojevic, 1992). Overall, in about 70% of cases there is a correspondence between the parents' attachment representation (secure–autonomous, dismissing, preoccupied, unresolved) and the child's attachment classification (secure, insecure–avoidant, insecure–ambivalent, and disorganized). The correspondence is even higher (75%) if we differentiate only between the "secure" and "insecure" attachment categories (van IJzendoorn, 1995).

In these studies the quality of the children's attachment was evaluated separately with regard to their mothers and their fathers. The results varied; in some cases a secure attachment quality existed in relation to the mother and an insecure one in relation to the father, or vice versa. This means that children construct separate and independent attachment relationships with each parent and that these can be differentiated. However, across studies, the correspondence between the fathers' AAI classification and their children's attachment quality was found to be lower than with the mothers (van IJzendoorn & De Wolff, 1997).

Interestingly, parental AAI classifications proved to be a more reliable predictor of a child's attachment quality than was parental sensitivity measured behaviorally (Grossmann, Fremmor-Bombik, Rudolph, & Grossmann, 1998). This means that a mental structure in the parents— their state of mind vis-à-vis attachment—appears to affect the attachment quality of their children.

Many longitudinal studies have been carried out in an effort to answer questions about the development of attachment over the lifespan (e.g., Egeland and Sroufe in Minnesota; Grossmann and Grossmann in Germany; Sagi and colleagues in Israel). In Germany longitudinal studies were conducted on the development of normal full-term infants both in Bielefeld and in Regensburg (Grossmann et al., 1993). My research team in Ulm also conducted a longitudinal study of very small premature infants. Although the Ulm study has not yet been fully evaluated, studies of healthy full-term infants demonstrate that their attachment quality is relatively stable from 12 months to 5 years.

Many studies have shown moderate correlations between early attachment quality and children's behavior in the preschool. For example, Suess, Grossmann, and Sroufe (1992) found that children assessed as securely attached in infancy were characterized in preschool by their greater ability to find prosocial solutions to conflict situations than their insecurely attached peers. Along similar lines, secure 6-year-olds reacted to pictures that contain separation scenes (the Separation Anxiety Test) with solutions that suggest a secure attachment. Insecure children, on the other hand, did not talk about their own feelings about attachment, or they were so overwhelmed that they had difficulty finding appropriate solutions to the separation situations portrayed in the pictures. These results were first reported by Main and colleagues (1985) and replicated in Germany by Geiger (1991). These findings speak for a high level of stability of children's attachment organizations and relationships.

Correspondences were also found in follow-up assessments at age 10 with children from the Grossmann longitudinal studies. Children who were classified as securely attached at 12 months and whose mothers were classified as secure–autonomous on the basis of the AAI, reported that they sought out their parents in emotionally laden situations and in solving everyday problems more often than did insecurely attached children. These secure children were also more likely to say that they could count on parental support and draw on it in overwhelming situations. Additionally, they had a more realistic view of friendships and fewer conflicts with peers. One especially striking finding was that children whose attachment was characterized as insecure–avoidant at age 1 year mentioned negative feelings less often and were very reserved during the interview when emotionally laden subjects touching on their own feelings were brought up at 10 years (Scheuerer-Englisch, 1989). At this age too there were significant correlations between the mother's level of support for her children and her sensitivity in the first year.

Further longitudinal analyses from the German longitudinal studies have shown stability of attachment classifications from childhood to adolescence (Zimmermann et al., 1995). Although these studies found no stability when comparing attachment *quality* assessed at 12 months and attachment representation (AAI) at 16 years of age, there were correlations between adolescent and maternal attachment *representations*: 16-year-old adolescents with secure–autonomous AAIs tended to have mothers whose attachment representation had been classified as secure–autonomous when the adolescents were children. Analogous correlations were found for adolescents with insecure attachment representations.

Regarding fathers, Karin Grossmann (1997; Grossmann & Fremmer-Bombik, 1997) found that constructive and sensitive paternal play behavior (giving the child space and time to initiate, picking up on the child's suggestions, and, if necessary, giving emotional and manual support) was associated with secure–autonomous responses to the AAI when the children were 16 years old. However, there was no correlation between the adolescents' attachment representation (AAI) and the quality of their attachment to their fathers assessed in the Strange Situation in infancy. Grossmann therefore asked whether the father's sensitivity in the play interaction—that is, furthering the exploratory system—might be of greater importance to the development of a secure quality of attachment with him than his sensitivity when providing care.

Because more fathers are involved in caring for their infant children now than were a number of years ago, there is a need for a new set of studies to ascertain whether this correlation would obtain today, or whether fathers contribute to the development of attachment in their children in a different way.

All in all, these studies show that there are correlations between the attachment representation (AAIs) of the parents, their observable behavior in caregiving and interaction with their infants, and the later development of attachment quality in their children (e.g., Grossmann, Grossmann, & Zimmermann, 1999). However, despite significant continuities, changes in attachment patterns may be observed from the first year of life through adolescence, at both the behavioral and representational levels. Attachment during the first year of life, then, is not the sole determinant of future development, nor do infancy attachment classifications allow one to make absolute predictions. Other factors apparently exert a large influence, as shown by the following results from research into protective and risk factors (van IJzendoorn & Bakermans-Kranenburg, 1997).

## The Significance of Protective and Risk Factors

Because transgenerational research has shown that we cannot predict attachment patterns in the next generation with complete certainty, it may be assumed that various other external and internal factors influence the development of attachment quality positively or negatively. In other words, we must assume not a linear, but rather a multicausal, cyclical, or transactional model.

Current discussions revolve around the effect that interactional factors other than sensitivity as assessed by Ainsworth have on the child's development. These include synchronicity, reciprocity, rhythmicity, and the fine-tuning of the affective exchange in the early mother–infant interaction (for a review, see Stern, Hofer, Haft, & Dore, 1985), as well as somatic and social factors (Esser et al., 1996; Esser, Laucht, & Schmidt, 1995). The socioemotional development of attachment quality as assessed in the Strange Situation is only one aspect, albeit an important one, of the entire developmental spectrum of the parent–child relationship. This was already acknowledged by Ainsworth and colleagues (1978), who examined sensitivity at home across many areas, including play and socialization.

We may further conclude from longitudinal studies conducted by attachment researchers that important life events such as divorce, relocation, illness, or the death of a parent during the first year of life are capable of transforming a secure quality of attachment into an insecure one, and so these are to be viewed as risk factors (Becker-Stoll, 1997). In a study by Zimmermann and colleagues (1995; see also Grossmann et al., 1999), even adolescents who were evaluated as having a secure attachment to their mother at 1 year of age were very likely to have an insecure attachment representation (AAI) at 16 years if their parents had divorced.

Liotti (1992), who looked at the links between disorganized/disoriented behavior and dissociative symptoms, examined a group of patients some of whom had dissociative disorders. He found that 62%

of patients with dissociative symptoms had mothers who had lost an important attachment figure within 2 years of the patient's birth. Only 13% of patients without dissociative symptoms reported a similar loss.

Of course, a great deal depends on the extent to which secondary or tertiary attachment figures cushion the stress of critical life events, and support the child in overcoming it. Many studies of emotional stability and resilience in children conclude that the presence of at least *one* available attachment figure constitutes a protective factor and can prevent the child from decompensating in the face of stress and developing further symptoms. Under these conditions, the child's psyche may remain relatively healthy even in the face of great stress (see, e.g., Tress, 1986; Werner, 1990).

The potential protective influence of secondary attachment figures was also examined in a comprehensive study of over 1,000 children conducted in the United States by the National Institute of Child Health and Human Development (NICHD, 1994, 1996) who were seen with parents and in a variety of different childcare arrangements. The results with regard to the development of attachment indicate that the quality of nonfamilial care during early childhood can affect attachment quality, but only under certain circumstances. The risk of developing insecure attachment was particularly great for infants whose mothers were less sensitive, and whose quality of care outside the family was lower, who spent more hours per day in child daycare, and who experienced frequent shifts in care. However, if the mother was characteristically sensitive to her child's needs, then the daycare factors described above had no detectable deleterious effect. In other words, a child's secure attachment to his mother afforded a certain degree of protection. Evaluation of sex differences showed that boys reacted more adversely to stress factors than girls in the development of their attachment patterns. The results led the researchers to conclude that preventive measures should consistently concentrate on changing maternal influence factors.

Hédérvári (1995) examined separation anxiety in working and nonworking mothers. She found a statistical correlation between pronounced "generalized separation anxiety" in both working and nonworking mothers and insecure attachment in their children. These results led to the assumption that the mother's anxiety in the separation situation affects her behavior toward her child, and may have a greater effect on the development of her child's attachment than does the fact of her working. A similar study was undertaken in the United States by Hock and Schirtzinger (1992).

All in all, there are clear indications of a transactional process in the development of behavioral attachment patterns and attachment representations. Biologically determined factors such as the infant's irritability and temperament certainly play a role here (Sroufe, 1985). However, factors introduced by the parents, such as their own attachment strategies and the intellectual and behavioral characteristics that result from these strategies, are undoubtedly of greater significance. Social-influence factors such as the home environment and marital quality (Belsky, Rosenberger, & Crinic, 1995; Easterbrooks & Goldberg, 1984), as well as the parents' social support network (Crockenberg, 1981), still require much more probing study. Only in this way, as already proposed by Rutter (1972), will we be able to determine more precisely the interplay between protective and risk factors at the intrapsychic, behavioral, and interactional levels, as well as in the social context.

## Attachment and Separation in Other Psychotherapeutic Schools

Bowlby's attachment theory was certainly not the first theoretical treatment emphasizing the significance of attachment and separation— indeed, attachment theory itself developed out of psychoanalysis. Since most psychotherapeutic schools have their own ways of conceptualizing this significance, I will now summarize several different psychoanalytic theories and then review other psychological theories, as well.

### Psychodynamic Models

Sigmund Freud's original psychoanalytic formulations, which are based on drive theory, explain the development of attachment between mother and infant as a result of the satisfaction of the infant's oral and emotional needs through breast-feeding. Freud never supplied detailed information about whether oral needs must be satisfied by the mother in a sensitive way, or whether oral satisfaction supplied simply by the administration of nutrition and oral stimulation suffices for the formation of attachment. Libidinal oral satisfaction was seen as more important than the interactional quality of nursing (Freud, 1905/1953, p. 123; 1916–1917/1953).

Freud dealt with the significance of loss and separation in his groundbreaking work *Mourning and Melancholia* (1917/1963). He saw the grief phase that ensues after the loss of a loved one, along with the psychic grief work that is needed as a result, as psychodynamically grounded in our need to withdraw our emotional attachment and intrapsychic emotional "cathexis" to that person, so that we may then actually separate ourselves psychically, and therefore also emotionally, from him or her.

In his *Inhibitions, Symptoms and Anxiety* (1926/1959), Freud explained the separation anxiety experienced by the child when facing real impending loss of, or fantasized separation from, the mother. He assumed that the child becomes fearful when imagining that his "needs tension" will become much greater in the mother's absence, and that he will fall into a state of helplessness resulting from a feared absence of satisfaction.

According to Anna Freud (1958, 1960/1969), "the pleasure principle . . . is conceived as a principle which governs all mental activity in the immature and insufficiently structured personality. Since it embraces all mental processes, the tie to the mother is governed by it as well" (p. 176). As she conceived it, the infant's attachment to his mother occurs as a result of "the impact on the mind made by the acts of mothering, namely, with the pleasure–pain experiences which accompany primary instinctual reactions and form their mental content" (p. 170). She assumed "a first 'anaclitic' relationship to the mother, that is, a phase in which the pleasurable sensations derived from the gratification of major needs are instrumental in determining which person in the external world is selected for libidinal cathexis" (p. 176).

Anna Freud also presupposed that for the child to experience "the pain of separation," the child's cathexis of the mother must have achieved "object constancy" and that the child must have become somewhat independent of direct satisfaction of needs. If the mother is highly cathected with libido, separation from her will be experienced as extremely painful, and great longing will result. If the separation is of longer duration, an aggressive aspect, which exists in every relationship as ambivalence, will come to the fore. This results in a withdrawal of emotional cathexis, and even in a regression from the mental–symbolic level to the level of physical needs.

It is astonishing that, in spite of Sigmund Freud's fundamental early work in this field, theoretical work on the subject of separation, loss, and mourning took a backseat to sexuality in his psychoanalytic teachings, although he did talk about the relationship to the mother as the prototype for all later relationships in *An Outline of Psycho-Analysis* (1940/1964).

Anna Freud made comprehensive observations about the effects of separation and parent loss while caring for and treating children who had been left homeless and parentless by the war. In very detailed depictions, she and Dorothy Burlingham described the children's reactions to separation, not just from their parents, but from substitute attachment figures as well.[15] Anna Freud explained the reactions she observed in these children according to the framework provided by then-current psychoanalytic drive theory, and she rejected Bowlby's attachment-theory-based approach (A. Freud, 1980a, 1980b; A. Freud & Burlingham, 1944), although Bowlby (1969) later made use of these observations as evidence to support attachment theory.

René Spitz (1959), too, assumed that the infant lives in an undifferentiated psychic state after birth, during an "objectless stage" in which he does not experience his own body as separate from his surroundings. The "nourishing breast" is perceived as a part of himself.

Spitz (1959) described the child's "anaclitic [dependent] object choice," by which, as Sigmund Freud postulated, the infant becomes attached to the person who feeds, protects, and mothers him. The child's attachment to his mother results from the establishment of the psychic constancy of the libidinal object, which the infant achieves in the eighth month. Up until this time the infant makes his mother the preferred object of his libidinal satisfaction.

Spitz in 1935 was the first psychoanalyst to carry out direct and comprehensive observations of infants and the first to document these observations on film so that they could be evaluated later. His revolutionary studies of the effects of long-term separation from mothers upon infants in institutions ("total affective deprivation"), with all its negative consequences for the motor, cognitive, and emotional development of these children, led him to describe the phenomena of "hospitalism" and "anaclitic depression." Spitz was able to show that the complete developmental arrest observed in these children, which in some cases resulted in total physical and psychic collapse ("marasmus"), could be partially reversed after the mother's return. However, this was only possible so long as the separation had not lasted longer than 5 months and so long as the mother–child relationship *before* the separation had been satisfactory. This research on the effects of long-term separation between mother and infant, and on the consequences of "emotional starvation" of the infant in the absence of his mother's affective care, was a pioneering achievement. This work (in conjunction with Robertson and Bowlby's work) has fundamentally changed infant care and institutional child-care practices in many countries (Spitz, 1965).

D. W. Winnicott, who was a pediatrician and psychoanalyst and a proponent of object relations theory (trained by Melanie Klein), developed an interactional dyadic concept of the mother–child relationship, presumably based on his frequent observations of mothers and children. In object relations theory, the drive dynamic postulated by Freud is always seen in relation to a human being, an "object." Winnicott thus gave relationships an important role, but did not explicitly give up drive theory. He pointed out that observation of the infant without simultaneous direct or theoretical observation of the mother is impossible because without the mother "there is no such thing as a baby" (Winnicott, 1958). Winnicott postulated that, in order for the infant to develop an optimal feeling of self-worth, he has to see himself mirrored in his mother's affect. "Good enough mothering" (Winnicott, 1958) and the mother's "holding function" were deemed necessary for the development of attachment, in both the concrete and intrapsychic senses. His experience as a pediatrician led him to emphasize that environmental conditions could either promote or hinder the mother–child relationship (Winnicott, 1965).

Winnicott also introduced the concepts of the "transitional phenomena" and the "transitional object" (Winnicott, 1958). He had observed that children, if separated from their mothers, generally keep and cling to objects such as stuffed animals or blankets. His explanation for this behavior was that such preferred objects function as "transitional objects" and represent the absent mother. This enables the child to process the separation intrapsychically, and to bridge the transition from closeness to separation symbolically.[16]

In Edith Jacobson's (1978) ego psychology, the development of attachment is based on the formation of integrated self and object representations in the psyche of the infant and small child. During his early development, the infant must form a stable, reproducible, accessible representation of the self in the course of his many interactions with his mother. He must also develop a stable object representation of his most important attachment figure that can be activated and accessed psychically at any time, and cathected in an appropriate matter. This is how stable emotional relationships develop.

The infant is then no longer dependent on the actual presence of his mother. He has internalized her as an object representation, and can therefore separate from her. During the separation the mother, as fantasized object, does not disappear intrapsychically but rather remains accessible to recall as an object representation. This allows the infant to endure separation anxiety and fear of loss. Without object constancy, the infant experiences loss anxiety such that the mother is experienced as completely lost to the infant intrapsychically as soon as she is no longer visible. Later, when the small child has the beginnings of object constancy, separation anxiety results when separation actually occurs. The child fears that he cannot endure longer separation from his mother because he can only maintain object constancy for short periods of time. However, an infant can tolerate separation for a few minutes. With increasing object constancy, longer periods of separation may be tolerated without the inner image of the mother collapsing and the small child being overwhelmed by separation anxiety.

According to the theory put forward by Margaret Mahler (Mahler et al., 1975), the newborn infant initially lives in an autistic world until a close symbiosis between himself and his mother comes into being. During this phase the infant is psychically merged with his mother and has no intrapsychic boundaries.[17] From this initial symbiotic state, according to Mahler, the infant increasingly moves away from his mother through a process of individuation/separation. During this time he continually tests his capacity for autonomy and separateness from his mother, as well as engaging in rapprochement to her. Until he is approximately 2 or 3 years old and able to separate psychically as well as spatially from her in order to explore his surroundings, he must learn to tolerate emotional crises characterized by the ambivalence between his desire for autonomy and his need to be close to and dependent on his mother during the separations from her. Mahler called this phase the "rapprochement crisis."[18] She has given us an impressive description of how an infant who is in danger or does not yet have stable object constancy returns to the mother for short periods in order to "refuel" emotionally. This behavior in children can be observed quite nicely in her documentary films.

Fixations and disturbances may arise over the course of emerging from the initial close symbiotic relationship with the mother, which is bound up with the intrapsychic process of individuation and the development of identity.

In her theoretical work, Melanie Klein (1930, 1946) dealt primarily with early childhood fantasies, especially the significance of aggression and the death instinct, and with processes of projection and identification between infant and mother. According to this theory, the relationship between mother and child is from the beginning complicated by the fact that the infant is overwhelmed by a great number of aggressive and destructive fantasies that he can tame only with considerable help from intrapsychic splitting processes. For example, the infant fantasizes the mother who satisfies his needs as a "good mother," whereas the one who fails him and sets limits becomes the "bad mother"—as if the actual mother were split into different mother aspects. Klein referred to this phase as the "paranoid schizoid position." Only when the infant is psychically mature enough to be able to give up such splitting, and to integrate the good and bad images of the mother (so-called part objects) into a unitary image, will he be able to create boundaries between himself and his mother and become more independent of her. At this point, which Klein called the "depressive position," he can begin to detach from her.

For example, if the infant feels frustrated by his mother while trying to satisfy his needs, he becomes angry. The fantasies connected to this anger can become so overwhelmingly aggressive that he comes to feel internally separated from his mother and experiences anxiety. He also fears that his aggressive fantasies will destroy his representation of his mother, which consists of good and bad parts, and that he will therefore lose her. As a result of his increasing ability to experience loving feelings for the good part of his mother, he becomes able to re-create these feelings symbolically and store them intrapsychically. In this way, he is able to overcome his fear, his grief, and his feelings of despondency and hopelessness about the fantasized loss of the good mother— the reason this phase is called the "depressive position."

This process is promoted by the infant's growing ability to symbolize his mother. Interest in his surroundings grows as the child, at the peak of "oral ambivalence," wishes in his fantasies both to penetrate and to devour the good mother, which would destroy her. These fantasies generate fear, which is why the child's interests are ultimately transferred from the increasingly symbolized mother to his surroundings as a whole (Klein, 1930; Segal, 1983).[19]

Melanie Klein and Wilfred Bion claimed that the mother plays a crucial role in the success of this development because she must intrapsychically absorb the aggressive affects projected onto her by the infant, understand them, and then relate them back to the infant verbally and nonverbally in an acceptable, age-appropriate, and sensitive manner. Bion called this maternal capacity the "containment" function (1962).

Michael Balint (1969/1979) advanced object relations theory in notable ways with his concept of the "basic fault," a term that refers to a psychic fault from the preverbal phase of object relations as well as to his formulation of the new therapeutic beginning. He called the earliest form of object relationship "primary love"; in this phase, the mother–child relationship consists of a "harmonious mix-up" or a "harmonious interpenetrating mix-up" (Balint, 1969/1979, p. 200). He based his conception on Sándor Ferenczi, and like him determined that "the formal elements of the transference and the whole analytical situation derive from the parent–infant relationship" (Balint, 1961/1965a, p. 151). He saw "mutual interdependence" as particularly important for the parent–child relationship, in which the infant's libidinal satisfaction and the mother's must go hand in hand. Balint designated another type of relationship between mother and child—but also between adults—as "ocnophilia": the individual feels himself to be secure and protected from danger only when in the closest relation to another human being. Balint himself drew a parallel between his concept of ocnophilia and the attachment behavior described by Bowlby. He called the opposite behavior "philobatism." In this type of relationship, a human being seeks out "friendly expanses" so that he is able to hold other human beings at bay by spatial means. This description reminds us of the insecure–avoidant attachment pattern in attachment theory. Balint was aware that even a philobat had a great, although repressed, desire for relationship (Balint, 1959).

In order to successfully treat patients with a basic fault and create a new beginning, the therapist "should be willing to carry the patient, not actively but like water carries a swimmer or the earth carries the walker, that is, to be there for the patient, to be used without too much resistance against being used" (Balint, 1968/1979, p. 167). This formulation and some of his other ideas about technique are related to the concept of the "secure base" in attachment theory, which is seen as a necessary precondition for psychotherapeutic work. Indeed, Bowlby (1969) singles out Balint's work as influential in his formulation of attachment theory.

Heinz Kohut's self psychology (1971, 1971b) proceeds from the assumption that a so-called cohesive self develops within a matrix of empathic selfobjects. A selfobject is an object that carries out functions for the self that it is not able to carry out itself: the mother protects her infant from excessive stimuli because of his still-limited ability to regulate himself. The way in which the selfobject fulfills its functions—empathically or less so—becomes a part of the infant's experience of self and of self-worth. To this extent, the selfobject is experienced as a part of one's own self. Kohut differentiated among three important selfobject functions: the mirror function; the alter-ego or twinship function (which makes it possible for a child to feel he belongs to a "we"); and the function of the idealized parent imago. From the perspective of self psychology, the importance of the idealized parent imago (idealized selfobject) is to protect the infant's immature psyche from inundation by affects and other stimuli.

The similarity between the idealized parent imago and the principal attachment figure in attachment theory is particularly striking. If the child's attachment system is activated in a particular situation, as is demonstrated by seeking protection, and if the mother focuses in an empathic way on his external and intrapsychic needs, recognizes them, and picks up on and responds to them in a valuing way—in other words, satisfies them in an appropriate fashion without flooding the infant with stimuli—the child can feel secure and protected.

Later, the child will seek out ideals by means of which he experiences similar security and protection. Only when the selfobjects fulfill their phase-specific functions sufficiently well in close reciprocal interaction with the child will a mature cohesive self develop. If the functions of the selfobject were poorly carried out, the structure of the self will be more or less damaged.

There is another parallel between the concepts of self psychology and those of attachment theory: a self that has become "cohesive," like a secure self, can act as a protective factor in times of emotional stress. Under these circumstances an individual will be able to cope with separations and losses better than if he had not developed these qualities.

However, if the development of self is only partially successful and selfobject representations of important figures are unstable, separation from them may be experienced as a massive threat, which can lead to great narcissistic rage. This in turn may so threaten the self that it is in danger of fragmenting. In order to defend against this, the self attempts to achieve affect regulation by means of delusional grandiose fantasies, which might express themselves as follows: "I am absolutely independent of human relationships. I don't even need the person who abandoned me. In fact, that person is dependent on *me*."

If this defensive maneuver is unsuccessful, further regression may take place. This may lead to a massive crisis of self-worth with pronounced depressive feelings and auto-aggressive acts, which not infrequently result in self-injury (a child bangs his head against the wall until it bleeds, for example, or an adolescent causes a serious automobile accident) or suicide attempts (Henseler, 1974; Kohut, 1971b).

Köhler (1995) has pointed out how close to each other the concepts of "sensitivity" and Kohut's "empathy" really are. In her description of sensitivity, Ainsworth (see Ainsworth et al., 1974) proceeds from the idea that a mother's ability to understand her child's signals without distortion depends on her ability to feel and perceive the world from the infant's point of view. However, unlike empathy, the concept of sensitivity also contains the idea that the attachment figure must respond to the child appropriately and in a timely manner that is age-appropriate and does not frustrate the child. In my view, "appropriate," in this context, means that the reaction (in terms of the actual situation, the developmental stage, and cultural norms) has to be capable of triggering in the child an advance in development and maturation. Kohut describes empathy primarily in terms of an intrapsychic function, whereas "sensitivity" includes an action level as well, which is the result of empathic perception and processing.

Kohut's concept of empathy refers to a mode of perception on the part of the mother that relates to the intrapsychic condition of her infant. An attachment figure's "empathy" presupposes that she is able to differentiate the affect triggered in her by her child from her own affect, that is, to see it as coming from outside her and as the sole result of her affective resonance. In addition, her perception of affect should not be colored by her own pre-existing affects, nor should the child's emotional situation be changed by the mother's projection of her own affects (cf. Ainsworth et al., 1974; Köhler, 1998; Körner, 1998).

Daniel Stern (1986), unlike other psychoanalysts, constructed his theory on the basis of infant research and presumed the existence of an interactive exchange between infant and mother right from the outset. Stern proposed that during the preverbal stage of development subjective self-awareness develops in phases. Diverse and differentiated interactions, consisting of action patterns and affects, are the building blocks for the development of internal representations. Stern denies that there is an early autistic or symbiotic phase in the mother–child relationship and assumes that the mother–child relationship develops during the first year of life as a result of the interactions between them. "Representations of interactions that have been generalized," so-called RIGs (Stern, 1986, p. 143) from the mother–child relationship, are the building blocks for the development of an "internal working model," a term Stern borrowed from attachment theory.

According to the analytical psychology developed by Carl Gustav Jung, the infant develops from an undifferentiated matrix, the "Uroboros," an archetypal symbol of wholeness that includes the united primal parents as well as the state of undifferentiated chaos and the unconscious (Neumann, 1985). The infant's developmental path leads to an individuated and differentiated personality with autonomy and self-determination that necessitates psychic separation from the mother and father as well as from the corresponding archetypes.

Jacoby (1998) has connected Jung's theory of complexes with the results of modern infancy research in a remarkable way, pointing out how environmental conditions, dispositional factors, and interactional affective experiences with the primary attachment figure create psychic structures in the infant that can lead to corresponding complexes.

### The Learning Theory Model

Behavioral therapy, as far as I know, has not formulated a developmental explanation of attachment and separation behavior and the behavioral problems and disturbances that result from it. From the perspective of learning theory, however, it is relatively easy to explain how children regulate closeness and distance with important attachment figures from birth onward, as the result of such learning procedures as reinforcement or negative consequences (see also Bowlby, 1973). The mother signals to her infant precisely how much closeness or distance she wants by a multitude of minute interaction sequences; this process is transmitted, and presumably stored in the infant's memory, as affective–cognitive schemata.

The same thing occurs with regard to the infant's self-reliant and exploratory behavior. Here, as well, one can easily imagine that the mother reacts either encouragingly or anxiously to autonomous impulses from the child, who learns from this that separation is permitted up to a certain point, and that his mother either tolerates it or that nega-tive consequences result. The infant orients himself to his mother's be-havior and learns a behavioral model from her based on the extent to which she actually lives attachment, closeness, and distance in her rela-tionship.

In his conception of psychological therapy, Klaus Grawe (1998) also builds on Bowlby and describes attachment needs as an important determinant of experience and behavior that must be considered in gaining an understanding of how therapy accomplishes what it does. He embraces Bowlby's (1973) explanation of agoraphobia as a psychic dis-turbance of insecure–ambivalent attachment; he also accepts the results of studies carried out by Liotti (1991) that are based on the same expla-nation, and he describes an attachment-oriented approach to the treat-ment of patients with this specific disturbance (Grawe, 1998, pp. 115–121, 395–411).

The theoretical basis of interpersonal psychotherapy (Schramm, 1996) derives from both Bowlby and ideas put forward by Meyer (1957). It therefore embraces an explanatory developmental model based on attachment theory. This model gave rise to a therapeutic tech-nique specifically designed for the diagnosis and treatment of patients with depression. In the diagnosis and treatment of interpersonal prob-lems much value is placed on the therapeutic relationship, even though it is not regarded as a "transference relationship" in the psychoanalytic sense. Particularly in the treatment of depression, the therapist actively addresses as central themes the patient's past and current attachment re-lationships, including separations and losses.

### Models Based on Systems Theory

Some versions of systems theory claim, among other things, that visible and invisible attachments develop among individual members of a fam-ily, and that these control and regulate both the interactions among fam-ily members and the family equilibrium as a whole. Whether individua-tion is possible in such an attachment structure depends upon how the entire system comes to terms with the autonomy of an individual family member. If the development of autonomy in a child, or the announcement by an adolescent that he wants to leave home, threatens to destabilize the system as a whole (because certain psychopathologies in individual family members might become overt), the entire family may be inclined to insist on attachment loyalty, and either inhibit the child's separation impulses or prohibit them outright (Boszormenyi-Nagy & Spark, 1973; Cierpka, 1996; Stierlin, 1980).

## Summary

The foregoing remarks, which lay no claim to completeness, demonstrate that various psychological theories and psychotherapeutic schools have developed a variety of concepts regarding the formation and significance of attachments and the effect that separations may have on the mother–child relationship. Some of these theories contain certain parallels to or similarities to attachment theory; some of them relate explicitly to Bowlby. On the other hand, there are fundamental differences as well.

The differences between the psychodynamically oriented schools and attachment theory consist in this: that psychoanalysis is based on drive theory while attachment theory is based on behavioral–motivational systems, of which Bowlby specifically describes the attachment system. Furthermore, psychodynamic theories (except for Stern's theory) proceed from the idea that the mother–child relationship is characterized at the outset by an undifferentiated matrix in which psychic merging processes dominate. Self and object are fundamentally undifferentiated. Over the course of later development, intrapsychic self-representations and object representations in the child must be differentiated from this matrix, so that psychic boundaries and individuation are possible.

In Bowlby's conception, by contrast, the newborn does not perceive himself merged with his mother but rather is predisposed to be socially responsive (cf. also Stern, 1986). As a result, the attachment between infant and caregiver must *develop* during the first year of life, and is not a given, conditioned from the outset by the experience of symbiosis. A variety of attachment patterns may develop in the course of this interactional process.

# Section II

⁓

# Attachment Disorders

## ATTACHMENT AND PSYCHOPATHOLOGY

By 1973, when Bowlby published *Separation, Anxiety, and Anger*, he had already begun to consider the question whether there might be links between insecure attachment and particular psychopathologies. He was able to find evidence for such links between agoraphobia and insecure–ambivalent attachment. He also saw connections between insecure attachment patterns and various childhood phobias (animal phobias, for example) and came to understand school phobia in the context of either a child's or a parent's separation anxiety (see also Atkinson, 1997).[1]

During a growing number of longitudinal studies, some of them prospective, links emerged between insecure attachment and conduct disorders (such as antisocial behavior) in preschool- or school-age children (Greenberg, Cicchetti, & Cummings, 1990; Greenberg, DeKlyen, Endriga, & Speltz, 1997, 1991; Greenberg & Speltz, 1988). Greenberg interpreted these problem behaviors as a strategy for eliciting caregiving.

In connection with specific chronic diseases such as cystic fibrosis, Goldberg (1997) reported disproportionate numbers of children with insecure–disorganized attachment patterns. This was true also for children diagnosed with heart defects who had had heart surgery in early life. In addition, longitudinal studies have examined the development of attachment patterns in high-risk premature infants (see review by Buchheim, Brisch, & Kächele, 1999). The studies on premature infants yielded contradictory results. Some investigators found that the distribution of secure and insecure attachment patterns among premature infants resembled that observed among full-term infants (Easterbrooks, 1989; Goldberg, Corter, Lojkasek, & Minde, 1990; Goldberg, Perrotta, Minde, & Corter, 1986; Macey, Harmon, & Easterbrooks, 1987; Minde, Corter, & Goldberg, 1985; Rode, Chang, Nian, Fisch, & Sroufe, 1981), other researchers reported an increased incidence of insecure attachment in children who had been extremely premature (Berlin, 1991; Mangelsdorf et al., 1996; Minde, 1993a; Plunkett, Klein, & Meisels, 1988; Sajaniemi et al., 2001; Wille, 1991). Because of the unclear nature of the findings, we are looking at the development of attachment patterns in extremely small premature infants in our current prospective longitudinal study (Brisch et al., 1996), taking into consideration the neurobiological risk factors of prematurity, early parent–child interaction, and the parents' attachment's strategies (assessed with the AAI).

Studies also showed that children who were abused or neglected in early childhood more frequently exhibit insecure attachments than children who show no evidence of abuse (Cicchetti & Toth, 1995; Crittenden, 1985, 1995, 1997; Lyons-Ruth, Connell, & Zoll, 1989). Disorganized attachment patterns also occur disproportionately often in abused children (Carlson et al., 1989).

Infants with parents suffering from either depression (Cummings, 1990; Cummings & Cicchetti, 1990; Lyons-Ruth, Connell, Grunebaum, & Botein, 1990; Radke-Yarrow, 1991; Radke-Yarrow, Cummings, Kuczynski & Chapman, 1985) or schizophrenia (Naslund, Persson-Blennow, McNeal, Kaij, & Malmquist-Larsson, 1984) were examined in prospective longitudinal studies on the assumption that the parents' illness constituted a risk factor with regard to the development of their infants or young children's attachment to them. Despite somewhat inconsistent results, a consensus seems to be emerging that children from these high-risk groups of parents demonstrate a greater than expected incidence of insecure attachment. However, this may not become evident until age 2 or 3 (Spieker & Booth, 1988).

Additionally, a growing number of studies have uncovered links between infant attachment patterns and changes in physiological, immunological, and neurohormonal regulatory processes, raising the question of a possible connection between attachment patterns and psychosomatic illnesses (Hofer, 1995; Reite, 1990; Reite & Field, 1985). Cardiovascular processes with different reactions in change of heart rate were found in securely and insecurely attached infants. All infants react to separation with an increase in heart rate, but the highest level of change was found in insecurely attached and disorganized infants. Comparable results were found for changes in the endocrine system. For example, Spangler & Grossmann (1993) measured cortisol levels of infants before and after the Strange Situation and found that insecure–avoidant, insecure–ambivalent, and disorganized infants had a marked increase in the Strange Situation, whereas securely attached infants revealed a slight decrease. Results on changes in the immune system are not yet very clear, but they lead one to suspect that the secretory immunoglobulin sIgA is involved as well.

The results for insecure–avoidant infants are especially important for a possible understanding of the origin of psychosomatic diseases. Because insecure–avoidant infants showed marked physiological and endocrinological responses despite fewer behaviorally expressed stress reactions during the separation in the Strange Situation, it becomes clearer that the behavioral strategy of avoidant attached infants is not due to a variant of temperament but could be due to suppressed attachment behavior. The costs of a down-regulation in expression of affect and behavior are marked reactions of the regulatory systems. It is well known from psychosomatic patients that they neither feel nor express their affects openly, but have measurable stress reactions in their physiology and endocrinology. A high level of arousal in these regulatory systems, which is expressed neither in behavior nor in verbal communication, could predispose for the development of psychosomatic symptoms and diseases.

Insecure and, particularly, unresolved "states of mind" (assessed with the AAI) and disorganized attachment in infants or young children have been linked to borderline personality disorder (Fonagy et al., 1995), agoraphobia after traumatic sexual abuse in childhood (De Ruiter, 1994; De Ruiter & van IJzendoorn, 1992; Liotti, 1991), suicidal acting out in adolescents (Adam, Sheldon-Keller, & West, 1996, Lessard & Moretti, 1998), maternal depression (Cole-Detke & Kobak, 1994; Lyons-Ruth, Coennell, Grunebaum, & Botein, 1990; Murray & Cooper, 1997; Radke-Yarrow et al., 1985), vulnerability to psychiatric illnesses (Fonagy et al., 1996; Parkes, 1991; Pianta, Egeland, & Adam, 1996; Rogers, Ozonoff, & Maslin-Cole, 1991; Rosenstein & Horowitz, 1993; van IJzendoorn, 1995b), schizophrenics (Naslund et al, 1984) as well as forensic patients (Lamott et al., 1998), and patients with spasmodic torticollis (Scheidt et al., 1999).

Thus, an increasing number of studies indicate connections in various high-risk groups between an insecure attachment pattern in infancy or AAI classification in adulthood and mental disorders and symptoms. Because of its frequency in clinical samples, the disorganized attachment pattern in childhood appears to be of particular significance for the development of psychopathology. However, to date it has not been possible to link specific attachment patterns with specific psychopathologies, and, as far as I can tell, this is unlikely to occur. Instead, secure and insecure attachment should be seen respectively as protective and risk factors for the development of psychopathological symptoms; presumably, a secure attachment raises the threshold of vulnerability to stress while an insecure attachment lowers it.

Further research is essential to clarify these questions, and such research is currently being conducted in various clinics in Germany and elsewhere.

∿

## THE THEORY OF ATTACHMENT DISORDER

Both developmental psychologists and researchers studying developmental psychopathology point out that the original patterns of attachment identified by Mary Ainsworth (secure, avoidant, ambivalent) represent patterns of adaptation likely to be found in infants and parents from nonclinical populations. Accordingly, the avoidant attachment pattern, aspects of which remind a clinician of psychopathological behavior, is believed to represent a behavioral strategy by which children are able to adapt their attachment behavior to the attitudes of their parents. In this way, they can maintain a relationship with the parent although at a greater distance (Main & Weston, 1981). Because avoidantly attached children appear to know that signaling their desire for closeness will most likely be met with rejection, they learn, as early as the first year of life, to inhibit such attachment behaviors as protesting a separation, following, calling, crying, and clinging. Instead they hold themselves at a distance from the attachment figure, and in that way avoid being rebuffed. Attachment to the mother can be maintained, but at the cost of the child's desire for closeness. Among these children, avoidant behavior in attachment situations appears to be the best strategy for lessening the stress that rejection of attachment behavior elicits.

The behaviors subsumed under the category disorganized/disoriented by Main and Solomon (1990) cannot be viewed as an adaptive strategy, however. I suggest that the children who display them have *no* appropriate or adequate behavior pattern at their disposal in such stressful situations as separation and reunion. The disorganized/disoriented designation is given when infants (in the Strange Situation) exhibit contradictory behaviors that strike the outside observer as confusing (such as running part way to the mother, then stopping and running away; frozen movement; repetitive motor activity; etc.). These behaviors, which may last for only a few seconds, give the impression of a disturbed psychomotor state, and are reminiscent of some psychopathological behaviors found in dissociative states of patients with posttraumatic stress disorder. They are observed significantly more frequently in high-risk children who have had traumatic experiences. Main and her colleagues (Main, 1995; Main & Cassidy, 1988) discovered that these children tend to behave in a controlling fashion during reunions with a parent at age 6, displaying either a controlling–punitive or a controlling–caregiving response to the returning parent. In high-risk adults who have experienced unresolved loss or trauma it is more common than expected to find lapses of reasoning and discourse during the AAI. According to current insights, the child pattern is a relational state whereas the adult pattern may be a style or strategy for dealing with attachment thoughts and feelings in general.

In contrast, clinicians such as Fraiberg (1982), Lieberman and

Pawl (1988, 1990), and Zeanah, Mammen, and Lieberman (1993) had already noticed very different attachment patterns among groups of clinically ill children or children whose relationships with parents were highly disturbed. They saw these patterns as indicative of "attachment disorders." Work by Crittenden (1988, 1995) on abused and neglected children, too, led to an expansion of the original classification of attachment patterns in such children. She identified several distinctive behavior patterns in these high-risk children: one a mixture of inse-cure–avoidant and ambivalent attachment behavior, and another that contained an admixture of avoidance and disorganization. Main and Solomon (1990) also noticed some of these patterns and incorporated them into their "disorganized-disoriented" classification. That is, these researchers developed related but not identical concepts and descriptions for similar behavior patterns.

In extreme cases both groups described by Crittenden (1995) exhibited distorted affects and cognitions. Proceeding from her experience with high-risk groups, Crittenden also observed preschool-age children for behavioral idiosyncrasies such as compulsive caregiving behavior and overadaptation, both of which are related to the avoidant attachment pattern. Among the children with an ambivalent attachment pattern, she found a subgroup that exhibited aggressive threatening behavior and one that used helplessness as a behavioral strategy. She also added a punitive pattern for school-age children. Behaviors characteristic of this pattern ranged from threats and withdrawal in school-age children to paranoid behavior in adolescents. These extreme ways of behaving give rise to differing affective and cognitive deficits in children with avoidant and ambivalent attachment. According to Crittenden, avoidantly attached children use cognitive processes to defend against their affects, while affective processes in insecure–ambivalently attached children are so highly activated that they diminish cognitive abilities. Crittenden thus posited a fluid progression from attachment patterns that are still healthy to variants of attachment quality that border on psychopathology.

In all of the mother–child dyads in Crittenden's high-risk sample of preschool to school-age children, she found that the expected "goal-corrected partnership" (Bowlby, 1969) did not develop. Instead, psychopathological behaviors became more entrenched with increasing age. These behaviors were found not only in the primary relationship of these children and adolescents but also in their other relationships and daily interactions (Crittenden, 1995).

Lieberman and Pawl (1995) developed a comprehensive San Francisco Infant–Parent Program that focused on underprivileged families with additional social risk factors such as poverty, unemployment, and cramped housing conditions. They treated parent–child pairs during home visits, using a "psychotherapy in the kitchen" approach derived from Fraiberg (see Fraiberg, Adelson, & Shapiro, 1975). They sought these high-risk families out for treatment at home because they might not have been willing to seek and accept psychotherapeutic help at an institution. Observation of an extensive range of attachment disorders led Liebermann and Pawl (1990) to formulate a typology of child attachment disorders based on the belief that the predisposition for the development of attachment can be changed and distorted by external social influences or severe parental psychopathology to the point that it may no longer be recognizable as related to attachment issues by an outsider (Belsky & Russell, 1998).

Their observations and preliminary work brought attachment theory back to the place where Bowlby had initially started: to the study of serious clinical problems. It is important to point out that not only parental psychopathology but aggravating external social factors, as well, can play a considerable role in inhibiting the development of healthy attachment. This insight has given impetus to the combination of social work and parent–infant psychotherapy in the Infant–Parent Program.

Greenspan and Lieberman (1995a, 1995b) subsequently developed a framework of attachment and its disorders from birth to 36 months that describes an "attachment homeostasis" (the smooth functional balance between attachment and exploration) in each of the included age groups and particularly in the first months of life. Deviations from this attachment homeostasis are described as severe, moderate, or mild disturbances that either overactivate the attachment system (anxious ambivalent attachment), thereby inhibiting exploration, or promote excessive exploration at the cost of decreased (avoidant) attachment.

~

## ATTACHMENT CLASSIFICATION
## IN DIAGNOSTIC MANUALS

Current diagnostic systems for psychiatric and psychic disorders are inadequate for the classification of attachment disorders as forms of severe psychopathology. An examination of the ICD-8 through ICD-10 diagnostic manuals and of DSM III-IV makes clear that no adequate diagnostic classification is possible of the multiplicity and severity of attachment disorders that are consistently seen in clinical practice.

Although diagnosis of child emotional disturbances was not considered in ICD-8, ICD-9 included the following emotional disturbances specific to childhood and adolescence (313): anxiety and fearfulness (313.0), misery and unhappiness (313.1), sensitivity, shyness, and social withdrawal (313.2), and relationship problems (313.3).

ICD-10 differentiates between an "Inhibited type" (Type I F94.1) and a "Disinhibited type" (Type II F94.2) of Reactive Attachment Disorder of Infancy or Early Childhood. DSM-III-R (313.89) and DSM-IV (313.89) contain similar diagnostic categories.

Type I in ICD-10 describes children who are very reluctant to attach to adults and who react with ambivalence and fear to attachment figures (i.e., F94.1). In Type II (i.e., F94.2) we see the opposite clinical picture: a disinhibited promiscuous readiness to attach to the most varied kinds of figures. Both of these types of behavior are seen as a direct consequence of extreme emotional and/or physical neglect and abuse, or as a result of constant change in the person of the attachment figure.

There are other diagnoses in the ICD classification that implicitly relate to issues relevant to attachment such as "disturbances of social behavior in the absence of social bonds" (F91.1), "Separation Anxiety Disorder" (F93.0), and disorders with "sensitivity, shyness and social withdrawal" (313.2).

Attachment disturbances may be seen as disturbances of *emotional* regulation (see ICD-9). However, in ICD-10, attachment disorders are no longer listed under emotional disorders but rather under the category "Other Disorders of Infancy, Childhood, or Adolescence." Even though deprivation or severe injury from the milieu is assumed to be crucial etiologically (in contradistinction to ICD-9), any relationship to emotional disturbance has been lost.

In the *Multiaxialen Klassifikationssystem für psychische Störungen des Kindes- und Jugendalters* [Multiaxial classification system of childhood and adolescent psychological disturbances], developed by Remschmidt and Schmidt (1994), many stress factors potentially affecting the development of attachment are listed under "Assoziierte aktuelle abnorme psychosoziale Umstände (Fünfte Achse)" [Relevant associated abnormal psychosocial conditions (fifth axis)]. These include abnormal interfamilial relationships characterized by a lack of warmth in the parent–child relationship, hostile rejection of the child with physical or sexual abuse, and disharmony between adults in the family. Other risk factors are psychiatric disturbance or deviant behavior in one of the parents; inadequate or distorted interfamilial communications; abnormal conditions of upbringing (including both excessive parental care and inadequate parental supervision and guidance) as well as abnormal immediate surroundings, institutional upbringing, loss of a loving attachment figure, threatening circumstances resulting from boarding the child with strangers, negatively changed family relationships resulting from a new family member, events that may lead to a decreased sense of self-worth, sexual abuse, and immediate anxiety-provoking experiences (pp. 147–154). In addition, events relevant to attachment such as "persecution or discrimination" and "migration and involuntary social transplantation" are listed under "social risk factors" (p. 156). These events have in common the potential to lead to severe impairment of the child's experience of attachment and relationship.

The *Diagnostic Classification: Zero to Three* (DC: 0–3; Zero to Three, 1994), which was developed specifically for infants and small children, also lists "Anxiety Disorders," "Prolonged Bereavement/Grief Reaction," "Depression," and "Mixed Disorder of Emotional Expressiveness" under affective disturbances (diagnostic categories 201–204) as well as "Reactive Attachment Deprivation/Maltreatment Disorder of Infancy and Early Childhood" (diagnostic category 206), all of which are manifested in the context of deprivation and abuse. The cause is assumed to be long-term neglect and abuse by the parents, so pronounced as to undermine the child's fundamental feeling of attachment security. The physical and emotional availability of the parents may be so insubstantial and unreliable (in cases of depression, for example, or drug abuse) that it is impossible for the child to construct an attachment to any single caregiver. Stressful environmental conditions such as constant changes in caregivers and long-term institutionalization or hospitalization can also impair the development of a secure attachment relationship.

Not one of the diagnostic systems described above contains an overarching explanatory model for a diagnosis of attachment disorders based on observed behavior and on social risk factors. This is all the more astonishing because some years ago typologies of attachment disorders based on attachment theory were described; however, to date attachment theory itself has not found its way into any of the extant classification systems to any great extent. In the following section I will describe a classification system for attachment disorders that I believe to be suitable for clinical use and that represents a first step toward a more differentiated diagnosis of attachment disorders.

~

## THE DIAGNOSIS AND TYPOLOGY
## OF ATTACHMENT DISORDERS

A point of principle to be made at the outset is that the diagnosis of attachment disorders cannot be based on the presence of insecure (avoidant and ambivalent) attachment patterns as described by Ainsworth and colleagues (1978). These attachment classifications are viewed as falling within the normal range of adaptive patterns, although they are considered to be risk factors in a child's further development, especially in the face of substantial stressors.

Rather, in children with an attachment disorder, one may observe very deviant patterns that are exhibited vis-à-vis a variety of attachment figures. These behaviors are not only situational; they may be observed as a stable pattern over long periods of time and in different contexts. It has been suggested that, before a diagnosis of attachment disorders can be made, these deviant behavior patterns must have been observed by different caregivers for a period of at least 6 months (Sameroff & Emde, 1989; Zeanah & Emde, 1994).

The diagnostic classification of attachment disorders presented below integrates both interactional criteria and those pertinent to attachment (cf. also Lieberman & Pawl, 1988, 1993; Lieberman, Weston, & Pawl, 1991; Zeanah & Emde, 1994). It can be applied through infancy, childhood, and adolescence (Brisch, Buchheim, & Kächele, 1999).

## No Signs of Attachment Behavior

Children in this category are remarkable in that they demonstrate *absolutely* no attachment behavior toward anyone. It is particularly notable that, even in obviously dangerous situations that normally trigger attachment behavior such as proximity seeking, these children do not turn toward a preferred figure. In situations of separation, they do not react with protest, or they protest during separation from anyone, without differentiation. When they do exhibit prosocial behavior, which occurs rather seldom, they do not prefer one figure over another, something that children with secure attachment behavior do. Developmentally, this classification should only be considered after the eighth month, because it is only after the development of stranger anxiety, which occurs at approximately 8 months of age, that one expects to find pronounced differentiation and preference for a principal attachment figure. This behavioral pattern is sometimes seen in children who have experienced numerous relational breaks and shifts during infancy or were brought up in institutions or multiple foster homes.

The behavior of children with this disorder is reminiscent of autism, but other characteristics of autism such as avoidance of physical contact, repetitive stereotypic behavior, and retardation of language development are not found here. This pattern of attachment disorder also reminds one of the classification of insecure–avoidant attachment described by Ainsworth and her colleagues (1978) in the Strange Situation. However, it is characteristic of this disorder that the absolutely avoidant attachment behavior of any person is expressed in an extreme

form, and additionally may include such peculiar and contradictory behaviors as undifferentiated protest on separation.

Children with an insecure–avoidant attachment pattern differ from
the unattached category in that they *do* form an attachment to a primary
attachment figure. They are oriented toward their attachment figures
even though they do not readily express missing them after a separation. The change in physiological stress, measured after separation, is
one indication of this attachment. Children with the attachment disorder described above, however, never establish a stable, reliable attachment, not even an insecure one. There is no attachment figure whom
they consider of particular importance as a safe haven, or whom they
seek out for protection when frightened or in danger.

## Undifferentiated Attachment Behavior

Children in this category behave in a friendly manner toward everyone
and do not differentiate between strangers and people they have known
for a long time, a behavior also called *social promiscuity*. These children
lack the usual shy and cautious reserve vis-à-vis strangers that is characteristic of small children whose attachment is not disturbed. These children do want to be consoled in stressful situations, but they will turn to
*any* person, even a complete stranger, who happens to be in the vicinity.
Yet they are rarely able to be consoled or calmed sufficiently to return,
for example, to playing.

A variation of this disorder has been called the *counterphobic*. These
children tend to endanger and injure themselves, and are frequently involved in accidents that on examination they appear to have courted by
their own flagrant risk-taking behavior (cf. Lieberman & Pawl, 1988).
This behavior cannot be explained away as simple curiosity or desire to
explore. These children completely forget about, or desist from, reassuring themselves in dangerous situations by glancing back at their attachment figure, the way securely attached children are known to do in anxiety-provoking situations. They lack the "social referencing" behavior
(Emde & Sorce, 1983) generally observed between infants and their
mothers during the first year. An exploring infant who encounters a
new situation that is unknown to him or that is fear-inducing will nor-

mally glance back at his attachment figure to reassure himself, by eye contact, about whether he should investigate this fear-inducing situation or whether exploratory behavior would be dangerous to him in some way. He reads his mother's nonverbal messages—her facial expressions or how she looks—and ascertains her "yes" or "no" to his further exploration. Children with this disorder also demonstrate a certain drivenness in their behavior. They apparently fail to learn from their painful accidents, and continue their high-risk behavior. These children are frequently brought by their parents to pediatric and surgical outpatient clinics for treatment. They persistently present with new injuries and often require emergency care. Both of these variants of attachment disorder (social promiscuity and high accident proneness) may be found in children in institutional or foster care whose attachment figures have changed frequently. They are also found in neglected children. It is important to consider the possibility of an attachment disorder in such children and then make an appropriate psychiatric diagnosis before beginning treatment.

Children with attention-deficit/hyperactivity disorder, whose exploratory behavior often appears to be driven and impulsive, differ from children with attachment disorders in that they do not generally have more frequent accidents than usual; their risk-taking behavior is not increased.

## Exaggerated Attachment Behavior[2]

This form of attachment disorder is characterized by excessive clinging: these children can be calmed and steadied only in close proximity to an attachment figure. In unfamiliar surroundings, in new situations, or when faced with a stranger, they react far more anxiously to a given trigger than one would expect, and they seek physical closeness to the attachment figure. For example, at school age they still want to be picked up and held, and stop exploring their surroundings or playing with interesting toys. Even when an attachment figure is holding them, they often appear anxiously tense and suspicious. They react to separation with excessive emotional distress; they cry, rage, and panic, and they are inconsolable. They resist even short separations violently, clinging to the attachment figure and protesting so loudly that separation may be prevented altogether. The attachment figure herself may avoid separations because she knows from experience exactly how violent the child's emotional reaction is apt to be.

This disorder may be observed in children whose mothers suffer from an extreme fear of loss. They need their children to serve as a secure emotional base for *them*, so they can stabilize themselves intrapsychically. These mothers, and very rarely fathers, are panicked by independent behavior in their children, and sometimes even by momentary separations. Whereas ambivalently attached children also cling, they do not show the extremely exaggerated behavior characteristic of this disorder.

## Inhibited Attachment Behavior

In contrast to the exaggerated attachment behavior described above, children with inhibited attachment behavior react to separation with little or no resistance. In interactions with attachment figures they appear inhibited and demonstrate *excessive compliance* (see also Crittenden, 1988). They usually respond to demands or orders from attachment figures immediately and without protest. Positive emotional exchanges with attachment figures appear limited. It is remarkable, however, that in the absence of a familiar attachment figure they are able to express their feelings freely and openly to strangers.

These children have learned, often as a result of extensive physical abuse or the use or threat of physical violence, to express their desire for attachment cautiously and reticently. Although they expect to find protection and safety, they fear that these may be delivered with threats of violence.

## Aggressive Attachment Behavior

Children exhibiting this attachment disorder organize their attachment relationships around physical and/or verbal aggression. This is their unmistakable way of expressing a desire for closeness to their attachment figure (see also Greenberg & Speltz, 1988).

Aggressive behavior in the service of relationship and contact is usually the prominent symptom and the reason why these children are often brought to psychiatric outpatient clinics in pediatric hospitals. Overt aggressive behavior among family members is common. This does not necessarily express itself in physical violence, but may show itself in other verbal and nonverbal ways. Family therapy sessions are often marked by a high level of aggressive tension that may not be recognized by family members or else be denied to outsiders.

In school and preschool these children are conspicuous as "troublemakers" and are often diagnosed as oppositional. These children and adolescents make initial contact in conspicuously aggressive interactions. They often calm down quickly when an attachment does start to develop, but this seldom occurs, as they are generally rejected by others because of their aggressive behavior. Their desire for attachment thus remains misunderstood. They must be distinguished from children with antisocial behavior problems in whom the symptoms of maladjustment are more generalized and not limited to aggressive interaction.

Bowlby (1973) pointed out that the rejection of a child's primary need for attachment that it is normally expressed in proximity seeking leads to aggression. The fear that an attachment relationship will not be formed, or that a developing relationship will be lost, leads via the experience of unassuaged attachment needs to a massive activation of attachment behavior and even to a battle for attachment. Because past experiences have led the child to expect rejection from the attachment figure, a desire for attachment may be primarily expressed by aggressive means.

## Attachment Behavior with Role Reversal

This type of attachment disorder is characterized by role reversal between the attachment figure and the child (parentification). The child is overly solicitous of the attachment figure and takes responsibility for the figure, substantially limiting his own exploration of his surroundings, or willingly foregoing it as soon as the attachment figure signals a need for help and support. A reversal of parent–child attachment roles has taken place. The child makes every effort to remain close to the attachment figure whether in familiar or unfamiliar surroundings. The child's demeanor is friendly, and he is overly solicitous and even controlling in his "shadowing" of the attachment figure. It is notable how unusually sensitive the child is to the other's well-being.

These children fear loss of the attachment figure as a result of, for example, suicide threats, actual attempted suicide, or imminent divorce. If they *have* in fact lost a parent to suicide, overly solicitous behavior with role reversal may be directed toward the remaining parent.

The behavior of these role-reversing children is superficially similar to that exhibited by securely attached children, whose sensitive behavior in a goal-corrected partnership allows them to perceive the needs of the attachment figure and respond to them in their behavior. However, if the child is securely attached, the interaction between mother and child is more intense and reciprocal, and this leads to the sort of positive development in the child that *promotes* exploration. In contrast, in the case of role reversed attachment disorders, parents do not reciprocate and answer the child's need for help or proximity. The difference is that the secure child who cares for the parent does not do so when in need of care him- or herself, and also does not do so compulsively.

## Psychosomatic Symptoms[3]

Attachment disturbances can also express themselves in psychosomatic symptoms. When the attachment figure displays a pronounced avoidant or distancing attitude toward the child, physical growth may slow down or even come to a halt, in spite of adequate physical care. The classic examples of this are nonorganic failure to thrive and hospitalism. Diagnostically, it is of great importance that emotional deprivation is not a phenomenon limited to the lower socioeconomic classes. It can occur at all social levels. Therapeutic work with the parents aims at a change in their emotional attitude toward the child. If this process is deemed to be moving too slowly, the child should be removed to another milieu, where the emotional care of the child is qualitatively better. The incipient development of attachment that results from such action affects physical growth, which will show gains after a period of standstill.

A principal attachment figure may react with excessive anxiety, paranoia, or even psychiatric illness, such as might result from postpartum depression or psychosis, at times of psychic overload. When this is accompanied by inconsistent care, with partial withdrawal and emotional unavailability during interactions (even though this does not necessarily entail physical neglect), an attachment disorder may result that far exceeds the anxious, clingy, and angry behavior seen in children with insecure–ambivalent attachment patterns. The child's anger is very great because the mother's behavior cannot be predicted. The mother's feelings for her child are overwhelmingly ambivalent. This affective tension in the relationship can lead to the formation of psychogenic symptoms, especially in infancy, including eating, crying, and sleep disorders (Brisch, 1998a; Minde, 1995; Naslund et al., 1984; Sroufe, 1979; Sroufe & Rutter, 1984).

When these mothers seek clinical help, they initially turn to the pediatrician. Differential diagnosis must exclude all physical causes, such as hormonal disturbances that could lead to growth retardation, or any organic causes of unusual crying, sleeping, and eating problems. However, if the pediatrician looks only for somatic causes and does not simultaneously pursue the possibility of an emotional cause (such as an attachment disorder), the necessary psychotherapeutic measures will not be undertaken. The symptoms can easily become chronic, which leads to increasing tension in the parent–child interaction—as in the case of a chronically irritable infant—so that symptoms become ingrained and possibly strengthened in a vicious cycle.

Occasionally mothers are seen during a postpregnancy checkup by a gynecologist who recognizes the mother's psychological illness. In this case, the physician should discuss with her potential difficulties with the infant.

In Germany the insights of attachment theory have to date been barely absorbed into the diagnostic thinking about adult patients, a situation that may be different in other countries (see also Dozier, Stovall, Albus, & Bates, 2001; Fonagy, 1998; Fonagy, Leigh, et al., 1996; Goldberg, Muir, & Kerr, 1995; Holmes, 1993, 1997; Sable, 2000; Sperling & Berman, 1994). It is unclear whether or not the categories of pathological attachment in children are valid for adults as well, although this can probably be assumed to be the case for some borderline patients. Their special psychopathology in behavior, self-reflective functioning, and defense processes remind the clinician of the behavioral pattern of disorganization (Fonagy et al., 1995; Fonagy, Steele, et al., 1996). It is also important to take into consideration that adult patients with attachment strategies or states of mind that are deemed insecure, but nonpathological in themselves (i.e., dismissing or preoccupied) may nevertheless not be able to find adequate solutions for severe problems encountered in certain life situations. Their attachment strategies are less flexible than those of secure ones, and hence they constitute a risk factor. It is also important to remember that even secure attachment strategies can break down if they do not lead to psychic balance or adaptation (Köhler, 1998).

Patients with disorganized attachment patterns (strategies or states of mind) certainly contribute in significant numbers to the clinical population, including especially dissociative illnesses, multiple personality disorders, and borderline disturbances. However, to date there are only a few reports on such illnesses and treatments and only a few initial studies (Liotti, 1992; Fonagy et al., 1995b; Fonagy, Leigh, et al., 1996; Fonagy et al., 1997).

# Section *III*

~

# Attachment Therapy

## THERAPEUTIC THEORY

Bowlby's theoretical ideas were an outgrowth of his practical experiences and observations. In the foreword to *A Secure Base: Clinical Implications of Attachment Theory* (Bowlby, 1988), he expressed regret that the theory he had developed for clinicians involved in the diagnosis and treatment of disturbed patients and families had been so little used in practice. In his opinion, use of the theory in practice was needed to extend our insight into the development of personality and psychopathology. Until then, his theory had mostly served to advance research in developmental psychology. Bowlby explained this disappointing reception of his theory by clinicians and their failure to apply it in practice by pointing out that the empirical, observationally based research on which he drew to formulate his theory struck some as too "behavioristic." Furthermore, he said, clinicians are busy people hesitant for that reason to commit time to try working with a new theory without first having concrete evidence that its translation into practice can further clinical understanding and therapeutic technique.

Psychoanalytic theory developed in the context of a treatment conceived as "one-person therapy" that is primarily centered on the patient. Even though Freud himself was relationally oriented and certainly worked interactionally, his vision of the psychoanalyst as a patient's "mirror" led his students and later psychoanalysts to emphasize a rather one-sided treatment relationship focused on the contributions of the patient rather than those of the analyst. Interactional reciprocity between patient and analyst was denied, at least theoretically. It took extensive discussion within the field of psychoanalysis before the ideas of object relations theoreticians, who called attention to the dyadic, interactive, and reciprocal processes between patient and therapist, gained greater prominence in treatment and in the training of candidates. To date, the disagreements within psychoanalysis regarding treatment focus have not been settled. Nevertheless, those who advocate an interactive approach have received much support from infant research. An infant is primed from the outset for interaction with a primary attachment figure, and nature has supplied the infant with an abundance of early capacities for perception and action. This is why we can say today that the relationship between mother and infant is reciprocal from the very beginning (Dornes, 1993, 1997). We must ascribe to infants an active capacity to contribute to the relationship. Bowlby was certainly one of the advocates of object relations theory who assumed an interactive relationship between mother and infant. For this reason, it seemed obvious to him that the therapeutic process and the therapeutic relationship should also be interactive and mutually established by the patient and the therapist. The idea that a psychoanalyst would limit himself to the role of mirror and abstain from active engagement in the relationship had no place in his conception (Köhler, 1995, 1998).

Comprehensive research on psychotherapeutic technique (Orlinsky, Grawe, & Parks, 1994) concluded that, of the wide array of variables that can influence the results of therapy, the therapeutic bond[1] between patient and therapist is of decisive predictive value. Research in psychotherapy shows a consistent connection between the quality of the therapeutic bond and the success of therapy. The "unspoken affective harmony" between patient and therapist and the "affective climate" are very important triggering factors in the creation and maintenance of therapeutic bonding. A good therapeutic bond affects the patient's readiness to open up and to break down defensive processes and resistance. The bond is deemed to have a primarily supportive quality. Establishing this bond is seen as a fundamental condition for the effective use of therapeutic techniques and the analysis of relational experiences. Especially when working with patients who have personality disorders and correspondingly severe psychopathology, the ability to establish and maintain a good therapeutic bond over the long term is a basic precondition for effective longer-term therapy. An open, consistent, and respectful attitude on the part of the therapist is particularly important for the creation of a therapeutic bond. These factors are very reminiscent of the basic therapeutic capacities and attitudes called for by client-centered therapy (Finke, 1994; Rogers, 1973).

These consistent findings of research on psychotherapy (Rudolf, Grande, & Porsch, 1988) show similarities to attachment theory, in which the creation of a bond between patient and therapist is fundamental (Bowlby, 1988).

The attachment that grows between mother and child during early development, as well as the need for exploration and the behavior linked to it, can be transferred to the therapeutic situation. It is important to be clear, however, that what takes place in the therapeutic situation is never an exact reenactment of what was experienced in the original situation. Rather, we are dealing with early experiences that are already altered by the experience of later events.

I assume that the patient's self- and object representations mature within the therapeutic relationship as a result of changes in affect, cognition, and behavior. According to Bowlby, the child's inner working model of self and attachment figure and the adult's attachment representation or attachment strategy may change as a result of new attachment relationships (Bowlby, 1969, 1973, 1980). A working model, as conceptualized by Bowlby, is based on the actual experiences of the self in interaction with attachment figures. Research has shown that children can develop different working models for mother and father (see also Buchheim, Brisch, & Kächele, 1998; Köhler, 1998). Furthermore, under some circumstances, a child may develop two contradictory working models of the same relationship. In this case, Bowlby (1980) proposes, one working model is accessible to consciousness, while the other is defensively excluded from awareness. The latter situation arises, for example, when parents ridicule a child's attachment behavior, but tell the child that their rejecting behavior is motivated by love.

In my clinical experience, an emphasis on attachment-related issues facilitates work with emotional disorders. Such a thematic focus could include issues related to attachment, separation, loss, and exploration. The concept of attachment can be viewed as a basic factor that affects all therapeutic methods and thus represents a basic precondition for psychotherapeutic work. Proceeding from the notion of the therapist as "secure base" (Bowlby, 1988), other seemingly unrelated aspects of emotional problems, such as disorders of drive dynamics or behavior, can be worked through either successively or in parallel.

Without a secure base—in other words, without a secure therapeutic attachment—it is difficult to work through affectively laden conflicts involving drive dynamics. Therapeutic work on drive conflicts can trigger considerable anxiety in the patient, who seeks a secure attachment figure in the therapist so that he can use that attachment to tolerate his anxiety. When the therapist as secure base is prepared to absorb this anxiety, conflicts may be processed. Without a secure base, the patient may be unable to endure the anxiety and fall back on resistance and defense. However, he will unconsciously continue to desire the establishment of a secure base with the therapist so that he can find the relational support that allows him to cope with his anxiety.

~

## TREATMENT TECHNIQUE

Bowlby dealt with the therapeutic application of attachment theory in various articles now collected in *A Secure Base: Clinical Implications of Attachment Theory* (Bowlby, 1988).

### General Considerations for Adult Psychotherapy

A patient seeking a therapist is generally anxious and fearful, and the therapist must expect, for this reason, that the patient's attachment system is activated to some extent. The patient will try to find someone to take the role of attachment figure by any means at his disposal, including means that have been distorted by his disorder. He focuses this search upon the therapist.

My experience with adult psychotherapy leads me to believe that the therapist must take the following points into consideration:

- In his caregiving behavior, the therapist must allow the help-seeking patient to speak to him via his activated attachment system, and make himself emotionally available to the patient. This includes budgeting sufficient time and space.
- The therapist must function as a reliable secure base from which the patient can safely work through his problems.[2]
- Taking the various attachment patterns into consideration, the therapist must be flexible in the way he handles closeness and distance with the patient, both in their interactions and in the establishment of the therapeutic setting.
- The therapist should encourage the patient to think about what attachment strategies he is presently using in his interactions with his important attachment figures.
- The therapist must urge the patient to examine the therapeutic relationship in detail. The therapist himself must do so, as well, because this is where all the perceptions of relationship conditioned by one's representations of one's parents and oneself are reflected.
- The patient should be cautiously encouraged to compare his current perceptions and feelings with those experienced in childhood.
- It should be made clear to the patient that his painful experiences with attachment and relationship, and the distorted representations of self and object that arose from these experiences, are probably inappropriate for dealing with current important relationships: in other words, that they are outdated.[3]
- In his careful dissolution of the therapeutic bond, the therapist serves as a model for dealing with separation. Separation is left to the patient's initiative, as a forced separation initiated by the therapist could be experienced as rejection. The patient should

be encouraged to verbalize his separation anxieties and his questions about being on his own without the therapist—perhaps even to do some experimenting. Physical separation is not the same as loss of the "secure base." Should the patient need help at a later date, he would still be able to rely on the therapist.

- A therapist who offers more closeness than the patient can handle (and which is therefore experienced as a threat) may trigger a premature desire for separation and/or more distance in the therapeutic relationship in patients with an avoidant pattern of attachment.

These aspects of therapeutic technique, grounded in interactional understanding, are based on the belief that early childhood interactions between attachment figures and child carry over to therapy. This ascribes to attachment processes a fundamental role in the creation of a therapeutic relationship, and is thus the central variable in the therapeutic process. Because patients with disordered social relationships generally do not bring a secure–autonomous strategy vis-à-vis attachment into their relationship with the therapist, it is the therapist's central task to become a secure base for the patient. This demands great sensitivity and empathy as the therapist adjusts to or feels his way into the patient's distorted attachment needs and the often bizarre interactional behaviors that arise from them. In this respect, child, adolescent, and adult therapies do not differ. The qualities Ainsworth called for—sensitivity in perceiving the patient's signals and the capacity to interpret them correctly and react to them appropriately and promptly—are just as necessary in the therapeutic situation and are just as helpful there as they are in the creation of attachment between mother and child.

Even when the patient's chief complaint, such as a sleep disturbance, appears not to be linked to relationship issues, constellations of relationships will quickly become associated with the symptom, and the therapist will recognize these as significant triggers or sustaining factors.

The discussion with patients of both current and childhood forms of important attachment relationships, which Bowlby recommended, will probably not just happen spontaneously in therapy. Although the patient comes to therapy with the more or less conscious intention of discussing problems and difficulties in interactional relationships, unconscious processes interfere with this desire because of anxiety-provoking themes and conflicts. This is precisely why the therapist's way of structuring the therapeutic relationship is so crucial.

Bowlby proceeded from the assumption that early-childhood representations of self and parents with their corresponding attachment and exploratory strategies are reactivated in the transference. Through a consideration of relationship experiences—particularly attachment relationship experiences—in therapy, the patient's earlier self and object representations can be analyzed and understood. In this sense, Bowlby is wholly a psychoanalyst and adherent of object relations theory. Even insensitive behaviors on the part of the therapist may at times have a healing effect if the patient responds to them and if the therapist takes them seriously as actual perceptions of the patient and does not fall prey to a defensive transference interpretation (cf. also Thomä & Kächele, 1985, pp. 64–82). In the latter case, the therapist denies the patient's perceptions that his (the therapist's) behaviors were insensitive by associating them instead with the patient's early childhood ways of experiencing. An opportunity is therefore missed to analyze the actual experience of attachment that resulted from the therapeutic interaction. Interpretations in which the patient's actual perception of an experienced injury is repudiated by the therapist's current behavior only serve to defend the therapist, whose self-esteem may be threatened by the patient's criticism. There is no doubt that such occurrences represent a great injury to the patient and probably weaken the therapeutic bond. They may even contribute to the termination of therapy because the patient's primary need for attachment has been rejected. In such a situation the patient may actually experience a repetition of his adverse early childhood attachment interactions.

Eventually treatment allows the patient to gain access to his painful attachment and relationship experiences, depending on the extent to which he can perceive his own affects, such as rage and grief. He experiences how these early childhood experiences promoted the development of rigid representations of self and object that to this day condition his relationships to other people through perceptual distortions, and the destructive interactions that result. In early childhood, Bowlby noted, such aggression develops when the child's needs for attachment or exploration are not adequately satisfied. This view is completely in accord with Parens's theory of aggression. On the one hand, Parens defines a beneficial, healthy aggression or assertiveness that aims at understanding the world and acting in it, an idea very close to a concept of exploration. On the other hand, he also defines a destructive aggression, which he considers to be caused by early childhood experiences of massive frustration (Parens, 1993b).

## General Considerations for Child and Adolescent Psychotherapy

Bowlby's guidelines must be modified for child psychotherapy as follows:

- The child therapist must function as a reliable emotional and physical base in his caring behavior so that a secure attachment relationship can develop in spite of the child's attachment disorder.
- The therapist facilitates play that promotes, both through direct interaction and observation of symbolic play, the depiction of material that relates to the child's experienced relationships with his attachment figures.
- The therapist interprets attachment-related interactions between himself and the child either verbally or by participating in symbolic play interactions.
- The therapist fosters emotional expression related to attachment issues that emerge in the transference and links them to past attachment experiences.
- The therapist promotes, through new security-providing attachment experiences, an environment in which the child can free himself from earlier destructive and insecure attachments and can develop a secure attachment in the context of therapy.

- The therapist must dissolve the therapeutic bond carefully so that it will serve as a model for handling separations. Separation should be initiated by the patient and/or his parents; this makes it much less likely that the child will experience it as a rejection on the part of the therapist. Physical separation is not the same as loss of the "secure base"; should the child or parents need help at a later date, they can still rely on the therapist.

In child psychotherapy it seems especially obvious that the therapist must establish a secure base for the child patient because the child is so much closer in time to the early childhood process. The younger the child, the more he relies on an actual attachment figure. The therapist must function even more compellingly as a secure base than for an adult. This pertains even to his physical presence. Here, too, sensitivity is of fundamental importance. Children are considerably more honest and direct than adults, who can enter into mostly cognitive pro forma relationships. If children's need for attachment is not responded to in therapy, however, and appropriately taken into consideration from the outset, therapy becomes impossible, or is terminated after only a few hours.

In child therapy the child's play behavior is focused on material relating to attachment, separation, and exploration. Depending on the age of the child and the therapist's therapeutic orientation, attachment-related play interactions between child and therapist can be addressed either by direct verbal communication or interpretively in the course of participatory play, and the child can to some extent be confronted with that material. The extent of the confrontation, or of direct verbal uncovering of attachment themes, depends on the age of the child and his cognitive capacities. In general, children can themselves address attachment experiences, in regard both to transference and to actually experienced past attachments. If these experiences are too charged with anxiety and aggression, however, one must in my opinion proceed very cautiously. A therapeutic bond that is not yet secure can be overburdened if the child is flooded by the affects connected with these experiences, and if these are interpreted and explained too early.

The attachment system is activated when a session ends, over weekends, and during vacations and illnesses. In child therapy children can take home toys from the therapeutic space during separations, and I consider these helpful as transitional objects (after Winnicott, 1958) that can stand in symbolically for the therapist and the therapeutic relationship. Some children ask to have postcards sent, as proof that the therapist as attachment figure has not been lost as a result of the separation.

Concurrent psychotherapy of parents or attachment figures plays an important role in the treatment of children. Because the child can only realize the advances he makes in therapy to the extent that the parents are able to understand and accept them, the therapist must inform the parents about the basic theory of psychotherapy, the therapeutic process, and any insights that arise as work progresses, as well as the specific treatment plan undertaken and the changes that they may expect to see in their child. More intensive individual or couples psychotherapy may also be undertaken with the parents, depending on their own psychopathology. In such cases, the same aspects of attachment must be considered as in adult therapy.

Therefore, the child therapist must enter into a positive therapeutic attachment (i.e., become a secure base) not only for the child but also for the parents. If the parents are disconcerted by the therapist's relationship to the child or changes in the child's symptoms, or if they feel that the therapist rejects them or they themselves reject him, treatment will eventually fail because the parents, out of fear, will incline toward termination of therapy. The therapist must also establish a secure emotional base for the parents, demonstrating great sensitivity for *their* attachment needs (which may well be very different for mother and father) so that they will be able to discuss their own traumas, injuries, and experiences of loss and separation during their concurrent therapeutic work. Moreover, the parents' attachment and exploratory needs within their own relationship will generally be of considerable importance. If these needs are not well integrated in their partnership, the desires and needs for attachment of the partners may be transferred to the child, who may then be forced into the role of ersatz partner. Similar transference desires may be projected onto the therapist.

## Special Considerations

In patients with attachment disorders, it is very important to acknowledge actual but defensively excluded needs for attachment, and not to interpret the patient's defensive behavior merely in terms of regression and resistance (Köhler, 1992). This means that therapists must understand the entire spectrum of attachment patterns. Only in this way will they be able to recognize relevant disordered attachment behaviors. In this connection, the therapist must pay special attention to the significance of real experiences of separation and loss.

Changes in attachment figures during the first years of life, as well as inconsistent and ambivalent caregiving on the part of the attachment figure, must also be considered, as they will have influenced the current attachment patterns of the patient.

An avoidant attachment disorder places great demands on therapists. They must deal with the attachment needs against which patients are defending and carefully interpret them, while at the same time paying heed to the need for distance conditioned by the patient's disorder. Satisfaction of defensively excluded attachment needs may therefore be bound up with an emotional closeness that is too much for the patient. This represents a potential threat to the therapeutic relationship and can lead to termination of therapy.

In treating patients with ambivalent attachment disorders, the therapist must pay attention not only to the reliability and predictability of his emotional presence, but also to the clarity and contextualizing structure of the therapeutic setting. The therapist must not activate the patient's attachment system unnecessarily, by changing the therapeutic arrangements (postponement or cancellation of therapy sessions, for example) or by starting therapy sessions late.

In general, patients expect that their need for attachment will not be satisfied in therapy either, and that sooner or later they will experience the disappointment of their desire for attachment. Offering only as much caregiving and emotional closeness as the patient himself can regulate has been shown to be effective; allowing the patient to negotiate the frequency of sessions with the therapist is one way of doing this.

Special attention must also be paid to situations relating to separation. These include the beginnings and ends of sessions as well as breaks in treatment for weekends, vacations, or illnesses. Termination of treatment, or its recommencement, are also significant. These are precisely the situations in which a patient's need for receiving care is activated and the affects that are triggered become accessible to processing.

In addition to the focus on attachment-related experiences, a second focus on the exploration side of the equation is necessary. A child's need to explore can be inhibited—even extremely distorted or disordered—by interaction with his mother and other important attachment figures during early childhood. One of the reasons for a disorder in exploratory behavior is a mother's insecure attachment strategy or "state of mind." A parent may "cling" to the child as a result of his or her own psychopathology. Parental anxieties may thus completely deny the child the possibility to explore.

The need to explore will also sooner or later be activated in the psychotherapeutic interaction. Therapists who do not recognize this need may well interpret the patient's exploratory behavior as resistance to working through issues—as acting out against, or as avoidance of, the transference relationship. Therapists who understand the connection between attachment and exploration will consider whether the patient's enjoyment of exploration might not be indicating the development of a secure-base relationship. He can then be supportive of this enjoyment in his patient and not interpret his behavior as a form of resistance or defense.

The spectrum of conceivable forms of exploration is great not only in children but also in adolescents and adults. It may include attending growth-promoting programs, whether individual, group, or a combination. However, trips, vacations, and breaks in therapy initiated by the patient for his own exploratory purposes may also be seen in this light. Arguing that these represent resistance to analysis, many therapists and schools of therapy demand that patients adjust their vacations to those of the therapist. Any deviation is interpreted as a form of resistance and is treated accordingly. While this may be so in individual cases, this approach sometimes overlooks the healthy aspect of the exploring patient. An attitude that allows the patient a certain amount of choice in structuring the therapeutic setting—changes in session frequency, breaks for vacations, and the like—may offer more potential for the analysis of the reciprocal relationship between attachment and exploration than a therapeutic setting that rigidly sets session frequency and rules. This way of proceeding has proved itself especially valuable in the treatment of adolescents, because their need for autonomous exploration, sometimes at the cost of the denial of attachment needs, is central in their therapy.

It is still unclear to me whether what is activated in therapy is a dominant working model of approaching attachment relations with other people, or whether what is activated in therapy is a specific working model of mother or father in childhood. Köhler (1998) assumes that a hierarchy of working models (from specific to general) is formed. However, I regard it as an open question whether, apart from the "dominant" working model, there might not also be a "recessive" one that reappears later in life. The possibility that a "healthier" attachment pattern might exist that had been pushed into the background is an important one for therapy, but has not been proposed by attachment theorists. If present, such relationship strategies could then be reactivated in therapy and would not have to be newly constructed within therapy (L. Köhler, personal communication). Other problems may occur when patients have constructed two contradictory working models of the same relationship,[4] only one of which is accessible to consciousness, as described by Bowlby (1980) and elaborated by Bretherton (1995, 1998) with regard to children who were subjected to highly rejecting or traumatizing interactions. From the point of view of attachment theory, it makes little sense to probe these patients' free associations before the inconsistencies of their thought processes and the causes thereof are worked through (cf. also Köhler, 1998).

The secure base offered by therapy makes possible an affective "new beginning" (Balint, 1968/1979), or a "corrective emotional experience" (Alexander & French, 1946). It is a fundamental prerequisite for the processing of old maladaptive attachment patterns.

It is still an open question to what extent a change toward a more secure attachment representation is effected through the therapeutic techniques. There have been very few studies examining whether or not an insecure or disorganized attachment strategy, assessed with the Adult

Attachment Interview, may be converted into a secure strategy—in other words, whether a secure "state of mind" with respect to attachment can be achieved later, possibly as a result of new corrective attachment experiences in the course of psychotherapy (cf. also Main's [1995] "earned secure") Treatment reports of therapies during which changes in the AAI were found seem to speak in favor of this, as do the treatment cases that follow (cf. also Fonagy, Leigh, et al., 1996).

# *Section IV*

❧

# Treatment Cases
# from Clinical Practice

Because attachment and attachment disorders are ongoing processes
that extend across the life span, I will organize my clinical examples
developmentally, beginning with symptoms experienced during pregnancy or even before conception, and continuing into infancy, childhood, adolescence, and adulthood. My primary focus is on mental
illness and the patient–therapist relationship from an attachment theory
perspective. Other psychodynamic explanations for the development of
these disorders are possible, as are other treatment approaches called for
by these different theoretical frameworks, and I will cite several examples of such alternative viewpoints.[1]

❧

## MANIFESTATIONS OF ATTACHMENT DISORDERS
## PRIOR TO CONCEPTION

### The Unfulfilled Desire for Pregnancy—
### Fear of Attachment to the Fantasized Child

Fear of a close bond with a fantasied child can be so great that pregnancy may fail to occur, even when the patient expresses an intense
desire for a child.

*Initial Presentation and Symptoms*

Mrs. A. telephones me for the first time and asks whether I have a psychotherapy slot open. She sounds urgent, and won't take no for an answer. It doesn't seem possible to talk with her then about the deeper reasons for her call, how to structure the therapy, or waiting time; she wants and expects an explicit and immediate "Yes!" or "No!" I give in to her insistence and offer her a time for our initial meeting.

A young woman, rather petite, with fashionably short hair and sportily dressed, appears for the first session. She immediately apologizes, but then launches into a list of questions that she has written down and that she wants me to answer.

The reason for her visit, she says, is her unfulfilled desire for a child. She has been suffering for 5 years over this—she really wants a child—but to date all medical efforts, including a number of hormone treatments and several in vitro fertilizations, have been unsuccessful. Now she is seeking psychotherapeutic help on the advice of her gynecologist, but she is very skeptical about it. I sense the skepticism clearly in her gestures and facial expressions, but at the same time I feel that she is making demands and putting a lot of pressure on me. A certain distance grows between us as a result of her behavior and the written questions; it is as if she wants to use my psychotherapeutic competence by peppering me with questions but does not want to enter into a relationship.

*Patient History*

Mrs. A. was 27. She reported in a very controlled manner and in great detail that she had greatly longed for child for the past 5 years. She had been married for 6 years, but she did not initially respond to my question about whether the marriage was a happy one. According to her, the relationship was unproblematic, and she and her husband shared their day-to-day lives equitably; her husband was employed in a technical profession and was reliable and "correct"; she had no complaints about him. Over the past 5 years she had made tremendous advances in her own career. She had worked her way into a leading position in her profession, and by her own reports filled it very competently and with great enjoyment. She was very lively during this part of the discussion, and it was apparent that she was dedicated "heart and soul" to her profession. However, she said, it wasn't a career that she had always wanted, but a child. She had poured all of her energy into her professional advancement out of her disappointment in the child realm; at least it gave her satisfaction and a feeling of success.

Mrs. A. was the youngest of three daughters. Her sisters were 4 and 6 years older than she. She had been a latecomer and hadn't really "fit in" with her mother's professional plans. Her mother had been a successful professional, too, and had placed the children with a variety of family child care providers from an early age so that she would not be "left behind" in her profession. Mrs. A.'s first provider, the one she "loved most," had re-entered the workforce when Mrs. A. was 3 years old. Mrs. A. was therefore placed in an all-day preschool. She still thinks fondly about this first daycare provider and enjoys visiting her on her birthday now and then. Mrs. A. described her relationship with her mother as "well functioning." The family was generally very structured and organized so that school, profession, household, and children could somehow be balanced. Her father was a "real pal" who took her along to sporting events. Sports had always been very important to her, and she won a number of prizes as a child. This was especially pleasing to her father.

She described preschool and school as "no problem." She claimed that it still annoyed her that, in spite of good initial grades in the gymnasium, "I only managed 10th grade.[2] Somehow when I reached puberty I got out of step." She often suffered from the feeling that she had "no solid group of friends." She envied her sisters because they were "firmly ensconced" in a large circle, and her relationship with them was superficial: "They were much older and lived in their own world." She met her present husband when she was 18, and they married early. She still particularly admires his self-assured sense of direction and reliability: "He knows what he wants." Problems relating to independence from parents, which she had observed in a number of her colleagues during her training, were completely foreign to her. Even as a child she had dreamed that "One day I will travel around the whole world." The idea that one might feel homesick in the process was completely foreign to her too.

*Consideration of Attachment Dynamics*

It is not clear whether Mrs. A., the third daughter and "latecomer," had been a wanted child. Her most intense emotional relationship seems clearly to have been with her first daycare provider, with whom Mrs. A. is still in contact. From an attachment theory perspective, her relationship with her mother may be described as more or less distant to ambivalent. She seems to have had more of an emotional relationship with her father around their shared experience of sports and related achievement, in which she felt that her self-worth was recognized. But as a whole she described her relationship with her parents and sisters as "functional," that is, structured and organized around clear rules and expectations. It is doubtful that Mrs. A. was ever able to create a secure emotional base with her mother, her father, or her sisters. Her early development was focused around achievement. Exploration, rather than emotional attachment, was placed in the foreground. However, the patient suffered from loneliness and a lack of close friends and attachments at a time when puberty was increasing her need for autonomy. In the end, she was unable to live up to the precept "exploration instead of attachment." The result was school failure and graduation with a mid-level certificate that was presumably below her intellectual capacities.

The patient was eventually able to stabilize herself in the context of her relationship with the man who became her husband; he was able to transmit clarity, structure, and to some extent emotional security to her, and he also functioned as a reliable base. With this stability she has been able to advance in her profession to an astonishing degree, given her youth. Her choice of social work as a career may also be understood as a reaction formation that allowed her to live out her own emotional desires and her own needs for early care, emotional nourishment, protection, and safety.

Even at the beginning of her marriage the patient wavered between two very intense desires: for children and for professional self-actualization. In her effort to "make a child" she made use of all available means and techniques, with the more or less consistent cooperation of her husband. One gets the impression that "the art of the doable" is front and center, both in how she relates to reproductive medical specialists and to me during our initial consultation. She becomes very anxious at the prospect of entering emotionally into relationships that she cannot control by asking questions, doing something, or creating clear structures. Feelings of emptiness, grief, rage, or disappointment when something is not doable are mentioned almost as asides or are expressed in such a way that they can only be perceived in the countertransference.

I want to note, however, that what stands out in the countertransference initially is that the patient is under a great deal of pressure and wants to control the situation, the setting, and me in the service of her desire for a child. She is probably not at all conscious how much her overtly expressed desire to have a child betray's her own wish to relive and actualize her own desires for protection, safety, security, and a "secure emotional base." She describes her relationship to her husband as reflecting a "functional security." Her sexual relationship with him is not so much structured by spontaneous emotion as by her desire for children and by the calendar.

If I were to evaluate this patient from a more classical psychoanalytic perspective, I would understand her like this: The patient suffered considerable unfulfilled needs in her early relationship with her mother. Her father was the parent more available for attachment, and the actual emotionally caring mother in her life was her family childcare provider. The oedipal conflict had not been resolved, and she could gain her father's recognition only by achievement. She suffers from pronounced problems relating to self-worth and achievement that only partially defend against awareness of her unfulfilled emotional needs in early childhood. The area of "achievement" remains the most stable aspect of her personality, with generally good ego functions and excellent intellectual capacities. Her desire for children could be interpreted as an attempt to relive her early emotional needs. At the same time, she is afraid to get close to these early feelings of deprivation, rage, and disappointment. As a result, her desire for children is unconsciously ambivalent. In order to make this desire a reality, the patient would have to engage with her own early unfulfilled emotional needs; and in the end she would have to lavish on the child all of the emotional care and security that she yearns for herself.

In contrast, from the perspective of attachment dynamics, I would say that the patient was not able to use her biological parents as a secure base, nor did her relationship with her sisters act as a corrective. Her most secure emotional relationship was doubtless with her child care provider; however, this relationship ended abruptly when the patient was 3, and the provider decided to pursue her own career. This separation therefore resulted in another lasting disappointment. From a very early age, the patient was forced to "function" in her family. Achievement and independence were demanded, and were highly valued. This is especially apparent with regard to accomplishment in sports; in this context the patient and her father were able to relate emotionally, but she has never been able to experience real emotional security free from the demands of achievement. Her attachment pattern can be described as avoidant. Exploration and achievement are still very important to her, and they have led to a successful professional life. Her husband has been very important to her as well at the level of functional security, but she has had to ward off her desires for emotional security and being cared for. Her wish for children is an unconscious wish to reexperience secure emotional care, that is, the secure emotional base that she had lacked in childhood.

These early experiences, with all their ambivalence, can be expected to become active in the transference relationship. It is likely, too, that the patient will initially attempt to structure treatment along attachment–avoidant lines by signaling her wish for distance in spite of her desire for attachment, thereby "functionalizing" the therapeutic relationship.

*Therapy and Course*

Over the course of the first 25 sessions, the patient focused almost exclusively on her imagined fear that I really didn't want her as a patient. According to her, I had answered very hesitantly when she first called, and although I had set a time for an initial consultation, I had not given her a regular slot in my schedule. This preoccupation seemed to reflect her early fear of not being wanted. In contrast with my usual therapeutic practice, I told the patient that she was correct in her perception, that I had indeed initially had no firm slot for her. However, I added that in spite of this lack of time I had arranged an additional slot for her after we had met and I had become acquainted with her history. At one point, when I commented that her perception of me as distant on the phone might have been a repetition of her early relationship with her mother, she became pensive. It then became possible to talk about her early childhood, which had been ruled by her mother's professional strivings. It was only over the course of treatment, in the transference, that her own desires and needs for acceptance, protection, security, and caring, which reminded her of her early experiences with her child care provider, could be verbalized. This was followed by phases of deep grief, as well as rage and disappointment, over the fact that so many of her needs for closeness, which she had been able to experience for a few hours each day with the child care provider, could not be experienced equally with her own mother. With tears in her eyes, the patient admitted that she had always wished that her child care provider had been her natural mother. The evening separations when her own mother picked her up had been "a horror." She had longed deeply for her day care provider to put her to bed.

From the outset I allowed the patient to structure the therapeutic setting by presenting her with a number of different possibilities in terms of the intensity of therapy, ranging from an hour every other week, sitting, to 3 hours a week, lying down. She felt panicky at the idea of 3 hours of therapy a week, and agreed to come for an hour every 2 weeks, stressing repeatedly that I couldn't possibly have 3 hours a week for her anyway. The questions that we discussed in connection with the establishment of the treatment setting revolved around her trigger situation—the fear of not being wanted—and my emotional willingness to offer myself as a secure emotional base.

During the final third of her treatment, the patient was increasingly able to enter into the therapeutic relationship, and she expressed a desire to intensify the therapy, increasing it to three times a week. Although I was willing to comply with this wish, in fact I could not do so as quickly as the patient wanted. This led to a turbulent phase of aggressive quarreling, as it aroused earlier disappointments: mothers were never available when they were really needed. In working through this early rage, she became able to formulate the emotional need for attachment that she had directed toward her father. When she was a child, she had sought him out when her mother disappointed her. Only over time did it become clear to the patient how well she had been able to establish emotional closeness with her father in the context of achievement. She also realized for the first time that neither therapy nor conceiving a child can be understood from an achievement perspective. During this phase her relationship to her husband grew stronger. The couple planned a 4-week trip separate from their regular vacation time, to "really let ourselves be spoiled." Such independence from me can be viewed in terms of Margaret Mahler's individuation–separation. However, it is equally plausible to view this incipient new phase as a kind of exploration and as an emotional "entering into relationship with" her husband in the context of the secure emotional base provided by therapy. I received only short notice of this vacation, which had been booked before I learned about it. But although it did not accord at all well with my own plans, I readily acceded to the patient's wishes, due to my new understanding of the relationship between attachment and exploration. Earlier in my career I would have interpreted such behavior only as resistance and acting out, and I would have attempted to work it through based on that understanding.

On her return from this "very happy vacation," the patient decided that she wanted to reduce the frequency of our sessions; she wanted to spend more time with her husband and the new friends that she had made on the trip. The emotional relationship between her husband and herself, especially their sexual relationship, had intensified during their vacation. Though her original reason for coming to therapy, the desire for children, was still an unresolved issue, she wanted to terminate her treatment, which had now lasted for more than a year and a half, in 3 months. All in all, she had become considerably more able to establish contact and relationship; the depressive feelings, the experience of being empty inside and of functioning mechanically, had been resolved. Her relationship with her husband and with other important attachment figures and friends had deepened enough that the significance of the therapeutic relationship as a secure base had receded into the background. Perhaps because her internal working model had changed, the patient became aware of more opportunities to "get close to people"—

especially to her husband—and to "explore the world." At our final session, she said, "I can always call you again when I feel like it."

### Concluding Remarks and Follow-Up

Five months later I received an agitated call from the patient. She had just learned from her gynecologist that she was pregnant. Her greatest worry now was how to combine child and profession. She came to my office three times at monthly intervals for further conversations. In these discussions, her emotional acceptance of, and joy in, her child and her pregnancy were the primary topic, but also how she had managed to negotiate a partial reduction in her professional workload with her employer during the pregnancy, and was going to insist on arrangements to make things easier for herself after the child's birth. She did not want to end up in the same situation as her own mother, who, with the help of a child care provider, had to return to her old job immediately after expiration of her maternal leave. During these conversations, it became clear that the patient had become able to differentiate between her own attachment needs and the fantasied prenatal attachment needs of her child—"to focus emotionally completely on my child." She was also able to integrate her pronounced need for achievement, that is, exploration. I had the impression that the patient had become considerably more self-reflective and in touch with herself, and that she now looked upon me as a partner with whom she could discuss issues that she had thought about in advance of our sessions. No problems developed that would have required return to a therapeutic stance.

Transference was not "resolved" at the end of this therapy, as other therapeutic techniques prescribe; in contrast, a positive emotional attachment relationship was deliberately retained so that the patient would be able to call me again, as she did when she received the anxiety-provoking news of her pregnancy. What is conceptually new here is the idea of an intermittent treatment that supports the patient and in which certain aspects of her intense early feelings—especially those linked to unfulfilled attachment needs—are worked through.

This approach leaves open the possibility that, if unforeseen anxiety-provoking situations recur from time to time, the patient might avail herself of the therapist and the therapeutic situation as a secure base for counseling or short-term therapy.

~

# PRENATAL ATTACHMENT DISORDERS

## The Pregnant Mother's Fear That Imminent Birth May Dissolve Her Attachment to the Child

The emotional processes of the last trimester of pregnancy, and also the birth itself, demand that the mother-to-be prepare herself for a clear recognition of her child as a separate individual. A pregnant woman's fear of giving birth, which means separation from her child, can make the end of pregnancy difficult and complicate the delivery.

The question of whether, or how, an attachment disorder that is activated during pregnancy can impair the fetus's attachment to the mother, and the consequences this might have for the pre- and postnatal mother–child relationship, is worthy of discussion (Janus, 1996). In the following cases, however, I will concentrate on the experiences of the pregnant mother herself, as this is what I have had access to in my own therapeutic work.

*Initial Presentation and Symptoms*

Mrs. B. is referred to me for psychotherapy by her gynecologist, who tells me that he is at his "wits' end with this hysterical patient." Mrs. B. has been calling almost daily, he says, and she involves him in endless conversations; she is also coming in during office hours, distressed and upset by some new "problem" that she has discovered. Painstaking check-ups have repeatedly demonstrated an uncomplicated pregnancy. The patient is now in her 30th week. The child's growth is completely normal, and, from the gynecologist's point of view, there is absolutely no reason for concern. But he feels responsible for Mrs. B.'s two previous first-trimester miscarriages. He had been tardy in noticing signs of threatening complications and premature contractions because he had not taken Mrs. B.'s complaints seriously, believing her statements to be exaggerated. As a result, he is letting himself get too easily entangled in

Mrs. B.'s complaints. He realizes that he is becoming increasingly annoyed with her and that it is hard for him to maintain a positive professional demeanor with her. He asks whether psychotherapy in conjunction with his medical treatment might be possible, so that he might lighten the burden this relationship imposes upon him.

Mrs. B. calls me to make an initial appointment. She leaves no doubt on the phone that she considers psychotherapy unnecessary; she does not feel motivated to come in because her problem is with her pregnancy, not with her mind.

At our first consultation I see a very well-groomed and attractive 35-year-old woman, whose 30-week pregnancy is clearly showing. She declines the armchair I offer her, preferring to sit on a straight chair, because with her large belly she feels "squished in." She is concerned about keeping the pregnancy and fears dire complications: a result of her two previous miscarriages. I argue that the most difficult and longest period of her pregnancy is already behind her and that she can look forward to the birth with equanimity, but she counters this with a forceful objection: "Being a man, you can't possibly imagine how important it is to me to get through the next 15 weeks of pregnancy without complications." When I confront her with her Freudian "slip" about how much time she has left, and point out that she has only about 10 weeks left, Mrs. B. reacts with visible irritation and tells me that she worries about giving birth prematurely. A friend of hers had given birth to her baby at 29 weeks, and this was a great shock for everybody. To date, however, there had been no problems with Mrs. B.'s pregnancy. I asked her how she imagined the birth and, even more concretely, whether she was anxious about it; she denies this vehemently. Instead she describes in detail the complications that had already occurred in the form of a "pulling in the lower abdomen," which she interprets as "impending contractions." Medical checkups had not been unequivocal. I rather quickly understand my colleague's countertransference, as all of my attempts to reassure and calm Mrs. B. get nowhere, and it slowly dawns on me that in fact it is a wish to continue her pregnancy that preoccupies her most. Every time I bring up the subject of the impending birth or suggest that most of the pregnancy is already behind her, she brusquely rebuffs my explanations. Throughout these conversations

Mrs. B. keeps both arms wrapped around her prominent abdomen. The image emerges of a mother–unborn child unit that wants to keep anything away from her belly that might induce separation or birth.

At our initial meeting, I was surely anything but a secure base for Mrs. B. I was much too directly focused on birth and the child as a separate individual—in my intervention and representations. Doubtless I failed in our first session to acknowledge sufficiently Mrs. B.'s need for an overly close relationship with her child, as well as the revival of attachment needs in her relation to her gynecologist as well as to me.

*Patient History*

Mrs. B. is the older by 17 months of two daughters. She says that she was very sheltered at home and that she always had a very "intimate" relationship with her mother. She felt "pulled back and forth" in her relationship to her father; she still grieves his premature loss when she was 15, in the midst of puberty, and still "wanting to do a lot of things with him." However, after an 8-month battle with cancer her father died. At the time, she felt abandoned.

On questioning she told me that her relationship with her younger sister was competitive. For her sister everything in life had been easier, she said; her sister was successful in everything she did, she already had three children, and she was happily married. As a child, the patient had often had a feeling that her mother preferred her sister and had taken more time to be with her. Even today, her mother spends a great deal of time with her sister's children, her grandchildren. During Mrs. B.'s pregnancy, scenes from her childhood have been bubbling up: images of wanting to be held by her mother and being rejected, because her mother was already holding the younger sister and two children were simply "too much." Nevertheless, the patient clung to her mother, and felt that she had been sent to preschool too early; she envied her younger sister, who had their mother all to herself for the entire morning.

Mrs. B. was very successful in school. She had finished her studies and achieved a stable professional position at the time she met her husband. She maintains that her 5 years of marriage have been happy and that her greatest wish is to have a child. From the outset, this pregnancy has been burdened by a great many anxieties, because 2 years earlier she had experienced two miscarriages in relatively quick succession. At this point she bursts into tears, and finds it very difficult to calm down. Under these circumstances it becomes gradually easier to take the stance of an attachment figure in relation to her. In the context of her grief for the losses she suffered as a result of her previous miscarriages, as well as through her description of her relationship to her mother, I can more clearly discern and feel her longings. Emotionally and conceptually Mrs. B. did not yet have room for an image of birth and her own imminent separation from the child. This pregnancy "could have been the most beautiful time of my life," she said, if only she had not continually been plagued by her insecurity about "premature contractions." Mrs. B. feels "well taken care of" by her husband, even though he was very tied up with his work; he was often away on business, leaving her to spend many evenings at home alone. However, she said, this was not as bad as it used to be, because now she always had her baby with her.

*Consideration of Attachment Dynamics*

I presume that Mrs. B. was forced into precocious independence much too early by the birth of her younger sister when she was only 17 months old. Evidently, it was hard for the mother to maintain a supportive attachment relationship with both children simultaneously. As a 2-year-old, the patient always found her mother's arms occupied by her younger sister, when she wanted and sought closeness. As a result, a very insecure–ambivalent attachment pattern seems to have developed that was characterized by a continued desire for closeness, but also by rage and disappointment triggered by the mother's rebuffs. It is not clear to what extent Mrs. B.'s father was available as an alternative secure base during this early period. The loss of her father during puberty, when she was still hopeful of much more interaction with him, should not be viewed simply from an oedipal perspective. Rather, this traumatic loss occurred during adolescence. Neither in early childhood nor in puberty was the patient therefore able to experience that individuation and autonomy are best supported by secure attachment to parents. In early childhood she had partially lost her mother, and during her adolescence she had to deal with the traumatic loss of her father.

Mrs. B.'s pregnancy is another intense attachment experience as, together with her child, she is attempting to establish a secure base for herself. Her constant anxiety about an impending premature birth may well have been due to her earlier miscarriages. For this reason it would be entirely understandable that the patient should fear difficulties and complications despite assurances to the contrary. Nevertheless, it is surprising that no number of check-ups and assurances by her gynecologist suffices to provide her with the sense of security that she wants. The patient imagines that she must shelter her child from the outside world and from other people in order to maintain their prenatal unity as long as possible.

Images of birth, in this patient, are accompanied by traumatic fantasies. Her feelings are highly ambivalent. Although she experiences intense attachment to her unborn child, this very attachment has activated feelings of rage and disappointment, both toward her mother and the child.

Furthermore, she may unconsciously be seeing her baby in the role of the younger sister, for whose needs the patient had to make room. She may well have experienced her sister's birth as an "emotional separation" from her mother and therefore as rejection, and may have transferred the resulting feelings of rage and disappointment to her child.

In my view, it will be necessary during therapy to focus on the patient's preoccupied attachment strategy, that is, on her simultaneous desire for closeness and for boundaries. All in all, this is a very complicated relationship structure. It will be important for me not to get irritated by her ambivalent behavior, but to establish a secure base from which the patient can work through her own early relationship to her mother, including the disappointment and rage connected with her younger sister. The loss of her father may later become another focus. Not until the patient can feel assured of her secure base will she be able to accept her child as a separate individual, something birth demands but that she still experiences as a threat. Otherwise, from an attachment theory perspective, there remains the concern that the patient will invert the attachment relationship and treat her child as her secure base, with the accompanying highly ambivalent feelings that could actually lead to birth complications.

*Therapy and Course*

We met twice a week in face-to-face psychotherapy. The patient always sat in the chair she had used at our initial consultation. She impressed me as a "pregnant Madonna," seated on her throne and entirely wrapped up in herself: mother and child, completely closed off from the outside world. During the first phase of treatment, she focused intensely on terrifying complications and the impending premature birth. She talked about preschool memories dating from after her sister's birth. In the context of her increasing ability to use me as a secure base, Mrs. B. was able to bring in a family album, pointing out to me how she was always merely standing next to her mother, while her sister sat on her mother's lap. The fact that the photos showed her as holding her father's hand created an opening that let us examine her attachment to her father, who seems to have been an important secondary attachment figure for the patient, in a relationship that was far more than oedipal.

During this period, Mrs. B. irritated me repeatedly with "surprise attack" phone calls she would make to urgently discuss something that had just occurred to her (see Brisch, 2000). She had become very interested in developing the story of her childhood in the context of her own motherhood, and she seemed to place increasingly exclusive demands on my time and accessibility. Initially I would try to put her off until our next session, but this met with little success. Given her rivalrous fantasies about my other patients (therapy siblings), Mrs. B. used the phone to snatch the emotional sustenance she believed she could not otherwise get. Only later did I come to understand her telephone calls—structured much like those to her gynecologist—in terms of "sibling rivalry vis-à-vis her sister." As she remembered, "It was never possible to get my mother to hold me, even for a short time, because my younger sister was always there."

As the delivery date approached, Mrs. B. became very annoyed that she couldn't reach me on weekends, evenings, and during short vacations. Only now was she able to work through her rage and ambivalence toward her mother, as well as her denial of the imminent separation of birth. The idea that her child was an independent being who would follow its own path of development after birth was alien to her. It required real grief work for her to be able to entertain the fantasies in which she and the child might explore the world together as two people.

The birth proceeded without major complications. Mrs. B. delivered a healthy girl. That her own mother took very good care of her after the birth moved her deeply. She was able to use this support, and her mother's interest in her new grandchild, to recapture something of the emotional caring that she had desired of her mother. Her husband was a good father and cared devotedly for his little daughter. With his help it became easier for Mrs. B. to share the child. Therapy continued after the baby's birth, but less intensively and at a frequency determined by the patient. She brought her little daughter to the sessions and showed her off proudly. When the baby was 9 months old, she began to crawl around and explore my office; we were able to talk about the connections between Mrs. B.'s desires for attachment and exploration when she was a child and her feelings for the baby. In watching her daughter, the patient was able to reconstruct her own childhood experiences. After working through her ambivalence toward her mother and her early rage and disappointment, it became possible for her to feel relatively unambivalent about entrusting the grandmother with babysitting for her little daughter, making it possible to take a few hours off to continue training in her own profession.

Mrs. B. terminated treatment after 32 sessions; between her child care responsibilities, her household chores, and her professional training, her schedule was full, and she no longer considered psychotherapy to be urgent.

As a result of her ambivalent attachment relationship with her mother, the structuring of my initial relationship with the patient was quite difficult, but in a relatively short period of time she processed enough aspects of her early attachment experiences to be able to accept the birth separation. Continued therapy after the baby's birth, now based on direct interaction with her daughter, made it possible for her to look at aspects of her own life history in a new light as she saw them mirrored in her daughter's development. There was no long-term working through of the oedipal conflict or of the loss of her father; nevertheless, transference aspects of these experiences, though not explicitly expressed or interpreted, were probably of great importance in Mrs. B.'s therapy.

### Concluding Remarks and Follow-Up

The patient did not call again. In this case, too, I chose to forgo resolution of the transference in the classical sense, because the possibility remained that Mrs. B. might later experience conflicts in connection with her lively little daughter's developing exploration and autonomy, and seek renewed consultations.

## Complications in Pregnancy and High-Risk Pregnancies

Complications during pregnancy, such as premature contractions and bleeding, may damage attachment processes between mother and child.

### Initial Presentation and Symptoms

Mrs. C. is brought to the emergency ward, her pregnancy imperiled by premature contractions and bleeding. According to the emergency care physician, Mrs. C. broke into tears upon admission, and I am therefore called to consult.

I visit Mrs. C. in her room. She is lying stiffly on her back in bed; she is not crying, but looking impassively at the ceiling. She does not seem to notice that I have come in. I sit beside her bed and tell her that the emergency care physician has told me about her situation and has asked me to provide psychotherapeutic care. Mrs. C. remains silent for a long time; she does not look me in the eye, and she appears to be in her own world. I inquire about her condition and how she feels. There is another long silence. Finally Mrs. C. begins to tell her story in a low voice and with a flushed face: she has had contractions and some occasional bleeding, and it is unclear whether her baby, in its 25th week, will survive. She glances over and over again at the drip bag, as if she considers it more important to her future than our conversation. She gives me the medical facts: this is her first pregnancy, and everything had been "normal" until a week ago. Her descriptions are curiously free of emotion; all I feel is a terrible tension in the countertransference. I myself have become very tense and agitated, and am torn between asking questions or remaining silent, and between enduring the situation or attempting a very structured psychiatrically-oriented case history. On questioning, Mrs. C. tells me that, although this pregnancy may have been wanted, it was not planned. Her husband wanted children, but she had felt unsure; children demand so much, and she was not certain that she was up to the task. When she learned that she was pregnant, she was "basically for it," but she was never really happy about it. Now she doesn't know whether to wish for a "good conclusion" to her pregnancy or to be happy at the possibility of its ending. She has experienced it as a considerable overload, both physically and emotionally. For the past 2 days her blood pressure has been high, and only barely contained by medication. My own internal tension is such that I find myself pushing my chair away from her bed, creating more distance between us. Obviously, I am having difficulty tolerating spatial closeness with this patient.

Our meeting lasts only 15 minutes, and I arrange a further visit for the afternoon. I consider the situation to be acute and extremely dangerous, which is why I decide on shorter but more frequent contacts with Mrs. C. She agrees with this suggestion, but I am very uncertain as to whether she really desires any sort of contact at all. For most of our conversation Mrs. C. looks at the ceiling or at her infusion, and only once appears to notice me momentarily out of the corner of her eye. When I get up to leave, however, Mrs. C. holds my hand for a long time and wants to know in exact detail when in the afternoon I will come back and how long our conversation will last, so that she can plan for it and not be out of her room for a medical exam. She will make sure the nurses and physicians take our appointment into consideration when they make their plans. All this surprises me greatly, and makes clear how intensely Mrs. C. must have absorbed our conversation and how important this other visit, which I now firm up, is to her.

*Patient History*

Mrs. C. was an only child. Her relationship to her parents is still of great importance to her; and she relies particularly on their advice when she has to make a decision. Her mother "took good care" of her all her life; she had been an at-home mother and had always been there for her. Her father was always "puttering around and making things," and he was involved in a number of local organizations. Mrs. C. lived her life mostly alone with her mother. When her father was out of the house, she and her mother could pretty much do as they pleased. When her father was home, however, they had to adapt to his narrower ideas of order and cleanliness.

Mrs. C. got to know her present husband, who is 5½ years older than she is, during her training, when she was 17. She married against her parents' wishes a year later. To this day she is not exactly sure how that decision got made; it was very hard for her to marry without her parents' explicit consent, and their opinions are still very important to her. She lives only a few kilometers from her parents, and she sees her mother almost daily. According to her, her parents thought that a pregnancy now (Mrs. C. is 23) would be too much too soon. They consider their daughter too young and too immature to be a mother.

Only later did I learn, in short snippets, that Mrs. C.'s childhood had been burdened by the fact that her mother often left the house for hours at a time, even at night, when her husband returned home drunk and their quarrels threatened to escalate. At those times Mrs. C. locked herself in her room and hoped that her mother would return. In the morning, everything usually appeared to have "simmered down." She was never able to talk about these mysterious quarrels, which occurred approximately once a month; this was "taboo."

In our conversations, which never last longer than 20 minutes, it feels to me as if Mrs. C. oscillates between rigid emotional stiffness, including withdrawn encapsulation, and a teary structurelessness, which impresses me as the flip side of her emotional rigidity. When she "falls apart," she needs a great deal of support and structure as well as reassurance from me; at those times she seeks closeness and asks for more time to talk, and I have a hard time maintaining the structure and schedule of our conversations.

### Consideration of Attachment Dynamics

In my contact with Mrs. C. I experience her tense agitation alternating with strong demand for closeness and structuring during times of emotional turmoil and tears. I presume that these affective breaks in our relatedness mirror the early attachment interaction between Mrs. C. and her mother, who alternated between being overnurturing–controlling (a pattern that continues to this day) and absent during the nighttime flights that caused her daughter much insecurity. Almost certainly, Mrs. C. experienced her relationship to her father as distant or threatening, especially insofar as she blamed his periods of alcohol abuse for breaks in her relationship with her mother, who was not available to her at precisely those moments when she fearfully locked herself in her room. It is to be expected that her father's threatening behavior activated attachment behavior and desire for proximity with her mother. However, Mrs. C. could not achieve this proximity because her mother ran away, undoubtedly leaving her with a tremendously increased activation of her attachment system. Unfortunately, Mrs. C.'s attachment needs during these times of extreme fear remained unassuaged.

Her marriage to the father of her child represented Mrs. C.'s first autonomous move, but was one that was and is accompanied by much anxiety. Mrs. C. is almost childishly dependent on her husband. Moreover, her relationship with her parents, especially with her mother, is characterized by anxious dependence. Separation–individuation, as described by Margaret Mahler (Mahler et al., 1975), or the ability to explore her own wishes, interests, and capabilities in the context of a secure attachment, has hardly been realized, despite her marriage and choice to have a child. Mrs. C.'s daily contact with her mother is characterized by pronounced emotional dependence on her when making decisions.

During times when Mrs. C. walls herself off from me emotionally and I can hardly reach her, I experience with her a pattern of interaction that reminds me of disorganized attachment patterns, especially when she exhibits her sudden affective oscillations and breaks. It is hard to imagine how she could accept a pregnancy, given her emotional background. Her feelings and actions are determined largely externally—that is, by others: her parents and her husband. She therefore does not know whether she wants to continue the pregnancy, or to terminate it before complications set in. Her entanglement with her mother, and their rapid swings between closeness and distance, already appear to be repeating themselves between herself and her as yet unborn child.

### Therapy and Course

I established a very structured and stable situation with Mrs. C. Initially, I visited her twice daily for about 20 minutes, once in the morning and once in the afternoon. After a week our relationship was sufficiently stable that we began to meet for about 40 minutes daily. We both agreed to a firm schedule, but it was not always possible to keep to it. The organization of her medical care often interfered with our plans. Frequently Mrs. C. was out of her room for some medical procedure when I arrived. Whenever that happened, I left a note telling her when I would come again, or I would try to reach her to make the appointment by phone. All aspects of the structure of the therapeutic situation were very important to her, and so were consistency in scheduling and oral agreements. Occasionally our sessions were interrupted by surprise visits from her husband or parents who, it seemed to me, "lay siege" to her bed. All attempts to get Mrs. C. to ask her visitors to leave so that we could continue our conversation went unheeded. Mrs. C. acted like a helpless child completely at the mercy of her parents, and seemed to me to have neither will nor opinions of her own. Her mother immediately took verbal control of these situations, stating that her daughter didn't need to talk to me anymore because she now had visitors. The parents were clearly resistant to my psychotherapeutic efforts; they seemed to believe that they needed to protect their daughter from me. Her husband, on the other hand, seemed to be relieved by my visits and supported our time to talk. He expressly said that he wanted psychotherapeutic care for his wife.

The entire term of treatment lasted only about 2 weeks; Mrs. C. gave birth during the 27th week of her pregnancy.

The medical effort to maintain her pregnancy failed as her general condition deteriorated to the point where Mrs. C. needed several days of treatment in the intensive care unit after the baby's birth. During this time her husband visited the baby in the pediatric intensive care unit, who was doing quite well under the circumstances. I saw Mrs. C. three more times in the ICU, and we spoke briefly each time. When she came back to the general medical ward, she told me in the presence of her parents that now that her child was born she did not need further psychotherapeutic help.

In spite of this patient's attachment strategies, which appeared to be fundamentally insecure with disorganized aspects, I did succeed transiently in establishing a therapeutic alliance during the last weeks of her pregnancy by maintaining a highly structured and consistent relationship. Her social surroundings, however (in particular the omnipresence of her parents), made it impossible to establish the long-term psychotherapy that she needed. I suspect that my work with her triggered so much anxiety in Mrs. C.'s parents, particularly in her mother, that it was they who insisted on termination of treatment.

The treatment of patients of this kind, who by classic diagnostic criteria manifest aspects of a borderline personality structure, is technically difficult, both in terms of management and in the handling of the countertransference. This is especially so because the breaks in affective contact demand considerable relational constancy on the part of the therapist and entail the risk that the therapist may respond unempathically. This might occur if the therapist prematurely terminates therapy or interprets the patient's initial rejection as his not being welcome. The patient was disconcerted and suspicious, expecting that I would leave her when she was most afraid in the same way that she had been left by her mother. Quite simply, further signals from the patient (setting up of appointments) demonstrated how necessary a very structured situation, marked by constancy and reliability, is for therapy in such cases. This made it possible to construct, at least during this 14-day treatment, a consistent relationship with the patient.

*Concluding Remarks and Follow-Up*

I later learned that Mrs. C. had a very hard time relating to her baby and that the father had made himself available as the primary attachment figure and was establishing good relational contact with the child. Mrs. C. rejected all renewed offers of psychotherapeutic help.

## The Diagnosis of Prenatal Abnormalities

Prenatal ultrasound examination during the first half of pregnancy is now routinely performed to screen for fetal abnormalities. Under some circumstances the technique itself, as well as the determination of fetal abnormalities, may trigger considerable anxiety in a pregnant mother and adversely influence the development of the prenatal relationship between her and her child (Brisch, 1998b; Brisch, Bemmerer-Mayer, Munz, & Kächele, 1998).

*Initial Presentation and Symptoms*

A gynecologist inquires whether I will accept a pregnant mother for outpatient treatment; during the 16th week of pregnancy an ultrasound examination has revealed a developmental kidney abnormality in her fetus. All attempts on the gynecologist's part to explain to the patient that an abnormality of this kind poses no threat to her child's life were useless; unexpectedly, the patient could not be reassured and asked, in tears, that he allow her to terminate the pregnancy. He told her that he could not understand why she would want this, and that he could not consider this circumstance an indication for ending the pregnancy. The patient agreed to get additional help some other way, including psychotherapeutic help, because the physician–patient relationship was very tense at the moment.

The 27-year-old patient arrives red-eyed for our initial appointment. She fights to maintain her composure, but begins to cry after her first few words. "Everything could have been so beautiful; now everything is finished." She had wanted a child so badly, and now she has to prepare herself for ending the pregnancy, because she "cannot live with a handicapped child." At a purely cognitive level, she is unable to hear my reiteration of her gynecologist's statement that this kidney abnormality is not life-threatening. Emotional relief is impossible. She sits before me crying as though she is already grieving the child's loss: as if she is convinced that the child is already lost. In reality, the course of her pregnancy is completely normal, and there is no cause for alarm as far as the rest of the child's growth and development are concerned. My impression of the patient is of a sad and despairing child who in her need looks for protection and help; she triggers in me corresponding countertransference feelings of support and generosity.

### Patient History

Mrs. D. describes herself as the "sunshine" of her parents' lives. They were a very happy family. She describes her mother as helpful, open, and generous, and her relationship with her father as engaged and loving. The patient has a brother, who is 2 years younger, with whom she still has an affectionate relationship. Even when they were children they had many interests and hobbies in common. She describes her entire childhood, her school years, and her years of professional training uniformly as consisting of ideal circumstances and loving relationships. Even when I questioned her more closely there was no hint of any break at any point in her idyllic life story. When asked to provide some concrete examples[3] of this "wonderful childhood," however, her examples were not substantial, but continued in this diffusely idealizing vein. In the end, the whole narrative came across as so "blank" that I wondered what had had to be "blanked out."

The patient described her husband in equally idealized terms: an attractive, handsome, professionally dedicated young man. With support from her parents, the couple were building their own home. They had wanted the pregnancy, and the baby was to be born just after the house was completed and they had moved in. The patient simply could not understand the fact of the child's abnormality because she had done everything possible to ensure that the pregnancy, the birth, and the child would be as ideal as her description of the rest of her life story.

There was no room in this story for unpleasantness, disappointment, or other such feelings.

By the patient's description, this abnormality was the very first real unpleasantness that she had experienced in her life. She could not believe that she would ever feel happiness with "*this* child." Yet, in her many fantasies and reflections about her "ideal child," she had already made emotional room for the child, and the thought of breaking off the pregnancy was very difficult for her, even though in our initial conversation she depicted it as the only possible solution.

*Consideration of Attachment Dynamics*

I suspected that even in her childhood, and perhaps throughout her entire life, Mrs. D. had been able to experience attachment and relationship with her parents only when everything was "ideal." She was forced to be—and perhaps she actually was—the "sunshine" of her parents' lives. The parents permitted her to use them as a secure base only when she was able to satisfy their expectations and conform to their image. I hypothesized that all "negative" feelings, behaviors, and thoughts— those that were "less than ideal"—were felt by the patient, and originally by the parents as well, as so injurious that the patient learned early on to deny them, creating a "false self." Her talents and her well-functioning ego had largely allowed Mrs. D. to maintain and live out this idealized image of herself and her parents. During our initial conversation, however, it feels to me that I am not making genuine direct interactional contact with the person sitting opposite me, but I am instead looking at a polished surface.

Because Mrs. D. did not feel accepted as a child, with all her many good characteristics as well as her negative feelings and shortcomings, it is now not possible for her to accept her *own* child's abnormality, or to continue the establishment of her attachment. She had wanted to present her parents with an ideal grandchild. Even so, her desire for attachment appears to be very strong, and she has already established a very intense prenatal parental attachment to the baby. For this reason, the very idea of breaking off the pregnancy triggers intense feelings of grief, and a reaction as if she herself were now being rejected and dismissed by her parents. In her identification with her child, it is actually she her-self who is not accepted and feeling rejected by her own parents, insofar as she cannot present them with her "ideal" child.

Some might see this as narcissistic with a pronounced disorder of self-esteem. From the perspective of attachment dynamics, however, it appears that the patient received security, protection, and support from her parents only when she presented herself to them as the ideal "sun-shine child" they expected. She fears rejection if she—or now her child, with whom she strongly identifies—does not fit this predetermined im-age. And she cannot imagine her parents as a secure base in the context of the anxiety-provoking diagnosis of the child's abnormality. She does-n't want to talk to her parents about these findings because in her fanta-sies she expects only rejection. She has established a similar pattern in her relationship with her husband. For this reason, she has subsumed all of her life plans and her development to date into this idealizing at-tachment pattern.

*Therapy and Course*

From the very beginning, the patient sought a great deal of sympathy and support, and it was not difficult to offer this while developing a se-cure base with her. Her fantasies were completely occupied with the loss of, and parting from, her child. During our first 20 sessions (twice weekly, face-to-face) my interventions focused on how and whether she could conceive of life with this child. She rejected such images as "com-pletely impossible." It became increasingly clear during this exploration that she feared that rejection would come primarily from her parents. Her husband, on the other hand, had been reconciled to living with this child since he and his wife had spoken with the gynecologist and re-ceived detailed information about the consequences of the abnormality. Their very different attitudes led to conflict between them, however, which the couple found very difficult to talk about. The patient became increasingly depressive and apathetic; she lay in bed for hours, incapa-ble of working, and she brooded about the impending termination of her pregnancy.

At that time, I sought to intensify treatment, and her reliance on me as a secure base, by offering her a third session per week. The patient readily and gratefully accepted this suggestion. With great effort, she eventually became able to talk about the rejection that she expected from her parents—or, sometimes, actually experienced—when she was not as ideal a daughter as they expected. She recalled many events and scenes in which her parents had threatened the withdrawal of care and relationship when she did not perfectly fulfill this or that expectation. This began with her early independence, toilet training, and school performance. All in all, attachment became organized around the achievement principle and a superficially bright storybook normality. In view of these childhood memories, it was not possible for the patient to get support and help from her parents in fear-arousing and threatening situations because, in general, this would have meant that something was not ideal. In "times of need" she always found herself very alone, depressed, and "deeply sad." She would retreat to her room or walk alone for hours in the forest to hide from her parents the need to cry. To the extent that these childhood experiences could be processed in therapy, the patient was increasingly able to enter into an emotional relationship with her husband. The high point of her therapy occurred when a very tense Mrs. D., her heart racing, told her parents about the baby's abnormality. Her parents were very skeptical and critical of the diagnosis, but they did not put pressure on their daughter as she had expected, nor did they press her to terminate the pregnancy. This relieved her tremendously, and made it increasingly possible for her to make room in imagination and fantasy for a life with this child. In this effort she felt supported both by her therapy and by her husband. Her growing ability to make emotional room for the child was further promoted by the baby's conspicuous movements and growth. Mrs. D. continued to worry that her parents would change their minds after the baby's birth, rejecting him and withdrawing as grandparents, but it was no longer in question that she and her husband wanted to make a life with this child and look toward the future.

In the context of her ongoing therapy, and supported by her husband, the patient also became able to make decisions about many details of the new house by herself, without consulting her parents and, by so doing, risking their "rejection."

The end of the pregnancy and the birth were largely uncomplicated. The couple was happy with their newborn son. The kidney
abnormality caused no functional problems, and so, according to her,
"to all appearances, everything went normally." The patient had changed
emotionally to the point where she could accept her child with his abnormality, "just as he is."

## Concluding Remarks and Follow-Up

Given the relatively short course of therapy, this severe attachment disorder, which manifested itself clinically as a disorder of self-esteem,
could not be definitively treated or resolved. However, the treatment did
cushion the acute crisis of the patient's massive depression so that she
could work through enough of her early history to be able to wholly accept both the pregnancy and the child, abnormality and all.

Along with the secure base provided by therapy, her relationship
with her husband as a significant attachment figure was helpful, and it
must be noted in this context that a therapist in the course of therapy
has to be able to take into account all of a patient's attachment relationships: the supporting (protective) ones as well as the obstructive ones.
He must think and feel through them empathically and work them into
his therapeutic relationship with the patient. It would be an overestima-
tion to believe that one can achieve and maintain developmental progress in cases of severe attachment disorder through the therapeutic relationship alone. Therapeutic work is easier when an attachment figure
with whom the patient has a supportive and secure relationship can also
support the therapy process. By the same token, destructive relationships in the patient's surroundings can be an impediment to therapy, opposing or disturbing the patient's reliance on the therapist as a secure
base, and even pressing for termination of therapy.

Once a secure therapeutic base has been established, it is an important task to encourage and support the patient in developing other secure attachment relationships outside the therapy context before terminating therapy. This makes it easier to let go of the therapeutic
attachment upon termination. A trustworthy secure base established by
the patient outside of therapy creates a protective factor for his or her
future development.

Mrs. D. visited me with her husband and child for a final session several weeks after the baby's birth. She was full of pride about the "not so ideal child" that just happened to be *her* child. After that meeting, I heard nothing further from her.

~

## POSTNATAL ATTACHMENT DISORDER

### The Mother with Postpartum Depression

Numerous surveys indicate that as many as 15–20% of mothers suffer from a more or less pronounced postpartum depression after the birth of a full-term infant. This is not to be confused with the so-called baby blues, fits of crying that occur during the first 10 days after birth. Postpartum depression is a severe psychiatric disturbance; it can seriously impair the relationship between mother and child, and therefore requires care.

*Initial Presentation and Symptoms*

Mrs. E. calls to make an appointment on the advice of her pediatrician. In a very pleasant voice she asks whether I have a free slot in my schedule; she inquires as to the whens, wheres, and hows of psychotherapy; and she wonders whether she is inquiring in the right place, given her "depressive feelings." Because her pediatrician had apparently recommended me highly to her, I felt a spontaneous positive transference to me over the telephone. We discussed the logistics of our first meeting very carefully, as the patient had four children: 4-, 5-, and 7-year-olds, and a 5-month-old baby. We finally found a time in the morning, when the older children were in school; the patient will bring the youngest child with her. She is very relieved at this, because she does not want to "needlessly inconvenience" her mother, who has helped her a great deal with child care over the past months.

Mrs. E. arrives for our first meeting with her 5-month-old son asleep in a baby carrier. She tells me that she suffered depressive moods during the first months after each of her children was born, which were diagnosed as "endogenous." They were treated with antidepressants and supportive conversation with the psychiatrist.

But things have been particularly bad after this birth. For the past 3 months, she has been so depressed that she has not been able to do her household chores in the morning. She feels overwhelmed at having to cook meals, get the children to school, and care for the infant. That is why she sought out the support of her mother, who has taken over for hours and sometimes days at a time, and even relieved her of a large part of her housework. Her medication is the same as before, and the other times she felt that things eased up after 4–6 weeks. This time, however, she is feeling that her depression is getting deeper from week to week. She can't understand this, as she had wanted a fourth child, and the hormonal changes to which her gynecologist had attributed the main problem should have resolved long ago. She is now seeking psychotherapy for the first time because she felt that her discussions with the psychiatrist had been helpful and a relief, even though she saw him for only a short time. She says that at times she feels that she is at the end of her rope, and all she can do is crawl into bed; at other times she gets fidgety and restless in the evening and feels that she has to prepare a thousand things for the next day, but that she just can't see the forest for the trees. When things are going well, she is able to organize the household and has everything under control. Her husband has some flexibility in his work hours, and he has been more available than ever recently, supporting her with the children and the house. Compared to the earlier births, she is working less, she says, and she feels very dissatisfied with herself for needing so much help and support from others.

*Patient History*

Mrs. E. comes from a large family with six children. She is the second-oldest. She has a sister 2 years older, a twin brother and sister 2 years younger, and sisters 5 and 7 years younger than she. In common with the older sister who was her "big role model," she began very early to help her mother take care of her younger siblings, and so she learned about housekeeping and child rearing in the natural course of things. Her mother was the calm and balanced support of the family, and because of the help she received from her two oldest children she always had time and energy for her younger ones; in time of need, the patient said, she lent an ear to all. The family had been very involved with a religious community, from which they could always get help and support when difficulties arose. The patient describes the family structure as a social support network, in which her mother functioned as a sort of "Earth Mother, a source of calmness and security." Her father had always functioned more as the "Secretary of State" in the family; that is, he was responsible for organizational matters and outside activities. Nevertheless, the children had a very good time with him during evening playtimes and on vacations. Mrs. E.'s fondest wish had always been to have a large family like her mother's and joyfully watch her children grow. At the age of 20, therefore, she found a partner who was not so dedicated to his work and ambitious that he would have no time left over for the family. She is in active contact with her parents, her brothers and sisters, and her other relatives, and she can count on help from parents and acquaintances at times of need or crisis. She is involved with her church as well, and does volunteer work as a way of "getting away from the family every once in a while."

Toward the end of our first meeting the baby woke up, and I observed how empathically Mrs. E. dedicated herself to him. He became increasingly agitated, and the patient asked whether she could nurse him before getting him into the car, as it was time for his next meal. Mother and child appeared to function as a harmonious unit. However, the patient reported that he often became agitated and whiny and difficult to soothe, especially when things were hectic at home. At those times she herself often felt practically apathetic; she didn't know what to do, and would wait eagerly for her husband to get home so that she could hand the baby over to him. Her sleep was often disturbed, as well; she thought this might be just because she was exhausted and overstressed. It surprised her that, although the help she got from outside did relieve her, it evoked "even worse feelings" of inadequacy, because she felt that her failures were thus openly displayed before her own and other peoples' eyes.

## Consideration of Attachment Dynamics

I suspect that even though Mrs. E. did experience her mother as a secure base and had developed a fairly secure attachment initially, she had experienced a lack of mothering after the birth of the twins. Very early, she had to help take care of her younger siblings, pushing her own desires for being mothered into the background. As a result, her attachment needs were not always assuaged. Instead, she served as a precocious secure base for her siblings.

A classical dynamic viewpoint might suggest that the patient's oral needs had not been adequately satisfied and that she had consequently confused "having a mother" with "being a mother" and started a large family of her own. The increasing demands of her own children, however, especially during their first year, placed a great burden on her own resources, which were limited by the unfulfilled needs of her early years, and postpartum depression resulted. Her fourth child so overtaxed her emotional resources that his birth left her with a particularly severe postpartum depression, in which she herself had to be taken care of by her social network.

From an attachment perspective, one might conclude that with four children, one a difficult infant, the patient had hit the limit of her ability to react appropriately and sensitively, despite the sensitive interaction with her infant that I observed. There was an increasing gap between her actual capacities and the great demands of her daily life. For how many children can she serve as a secure base, given that, unlike her mother, she does not have older children who are capable of serving as secure substitute mothers, relieving her of some of her responsibilities? The help that she received from the network of grandparents and other reference persons in the community initially gave her some physical and emotional relief. But it could not disperse the feelings of inadequacy evoked by the discrepancy she felt between her fundamental ability to relate to her infant as a secure base and the real demands placed on her, which she did not feel equal to confronting. The actual demands that her children made on her began to outpace her capacities, opening a widening gap that she could not close with her own resources. Her retreat into bed, which neither really relieved her nor allowed her to regroup, demonstrated that the patient's early unfulfilled attachment needs made it difficult for her to make use of the help she was offered, and thus to gain sufficient strength and support to come to terms with the demands made upon her. The balance between serving as an attachment figure and accepting support from others when needed collapsed at this point, and she began to experience the external offers of support as indicative of failure to live up to what was expected of her. I expected that the patient's standards for maternal reponsiveness were very high and that she would make similarly rigorous demands on me. I thought that Winnicott's idea of the "good enough mother" might be a relief to her.

*Therapy and Course*

Although Mrs. E. came to our first sessions with her little son, she "allowed" herself to attend subsequent sessions alone, as her mother was able to take the child. We spent a great deal of time working through her problem with "being able to take something for myself and not sharing it," that is, using the therapy session only for herself, in order to satisfy her own desires for support, safety, and security. She recalled how she had had to share her mother with her other siblings; there was really not much time left over for "one-on-one."

The broad spectrum of the patient's sensitivity was revealed in her reports about her children and family. She could describe precisely her children's development and perceptions, as well as the demands they made on her at different ages. It was no wonder, given this high level of reflectiveness and her high standards, that she had reached her limit. The new baby had aggravated the situation because, due either to his reactivity or to his rather difficult temperament, he now had a complete lock on her attention and sensitivity. As a result, she felt an increasing discrepancy between her real and ideal self, leading to a state of physical and mental exhaustion. For this reason, treatment focused on the idea that she should make time for herself that she did not have to "share" with anybody, not only in therapy, but in her relationship with her husband, with her individual children, and even with her mother. I had a countertransference impression that the patient was eventually able to enjoy being alone for her sessions because she was out of reach of her family; it was "an hour just for me when nobody calls for Mom."

After 3 months of psychotherapy, her depressive symptoms had completely disappeared, except for a few days during which the patient had been kept up all night by her teething infant, leaving her physically exhausted the next day. However, she was able to understand the cause and to differentiate it from her original depressive symptoms.

Symptomatically, things were going considerably better for her. With her little son's increasing mobility, she discontinued her weekly sessions because she did not want to leave her "rambunctious little fellow" with her aged mother as often as before. Nevertheless, it was still important for her to be able to schedule appointments as needed, "like little islands where I can refuel." Because of this, treatment stretched out over 2 years, but at longer intervals. For the last third of the treatment, the patient used the sessions in part to clarify current issues in her own life: how much of a burden she could still impose on her aging mother, for instance, and her guilt about doing it. But she also used the sessions to discuss this or that issue of child-rearing and development and to think about the development of her children in the quiet surroundings afforded by a sort of parenting consultation.

### Concluding Remarks and Follow-Up

Even a very secure initial attachment experience does not protect a person from subsequent stresses of life, such as the birth of siblings. However, a secure attachment allows for a quicker recovery when the external issue disappears, making reflection possible, and more quickly possible as well.

It remains an open question whether Mrs. E.'s depressive symptoms remitted spontaneously or improved as a result of psychotherapy or medication. The etiology of postpartum depression is still unclear, and a multifactor process involving endocrinology, neurotransmitter physiology, and psychodynamics is being investigated. The insights afforded by attachment theory provide one possible way of understanding this patient's situation and illness, and of treating it. It would be interesting to know whether the depression would recur after another birth; however, the patient decided as a result of her therapy that raising four children, and setting them on the proper path, is a sufficient achievement.

Mrs. E. calls me occasionally to discuss briefly some question or another about child-rearing. She uses these opportunities to acquire some support for herself, which I am pleased to provide. No depressions such as those that occurred after her last baby's birth have recurred to date.

## The Mother with Postpartum Psychosis

Even today, mothers in treatment for postpartum psychosis are usually separated from their infants when inpatient psychiatric treatment is required. Psychiatric clinics in Germany still lack "mother and baby" units that would allow for simultaneous admission of the sick mother and her infant. There are as yet very few provisions in Germany for inpatient care of mother and child together (Hartmann, 1997a, 1997b; Lanszik, 1997). I will now discuss the difficult attachment processes that take place under such circumstances between psychotic mothers and their children.

*Initial Presentation and Symptoms*

Mrs. F. is admitted for inpatient psychiatric treatment of an acute postpartum psychosis; her first child had been born 2 weeks previously. She arrives with her husband, who holds her hand as if she were a child while she looks anxiously around the unit. During the intake procedures she continues to look deeply fearful, and as though she feels threatened. She insists that her husband remain for the intake examination. She grasps his hand throughout, pulling her chair close to him and clearly seeking his protection. She wants him to tell her story.

According to him, the pregnancy and birth of their baby daughter had been normal and completely unremarkable. They had looked forward to the pregnancy and to the child, and at first both mother and child had been well. But even in the clinic, the nurses had noticed that his wife had occasionally been "unreliable" in caring for the baby; for example, she had gone to the hospital shop, leaving her infant alone in her room crying. During the rooming-in period there had always been other patients who had looked out for the baby, and at first no one was terribly concerned about this behavior.

When the father did confront his wife, she reacted evasively and then suddenly withdrew into silence. He experienced her as being very changed and withdrawn, and he was not able to establish emotional contact with her again. He, the other patients, and the nurses had also begun to notice that she increasingly treated the infant as if she were a doll, becoming involved with her when she felt like it but then abruptly laying her down for reasons that nobody could fathom. Only during the course of a conversation with the psychiatrist who was brought in for consultation, and whom Mrs. F. continued to see after her discharge, did it become clear that at certain times the thought came to her that she must kill her child. For this reason, she removed herself from the baby's vicinity for fear that she would not be able to control her impulses.

Mrs. F. listens apparently unmoved to her husband's report. I learned later that she had been treated with neuroleptics, which would explain in part her restricted affect and her facial immobility. Because her husband and relatives feared that she might neglect the baby, or give in to her impulsive fantasies, outpatient psychiatric treatment notwithstanding, inpatient care was finally advised. Mrs. F. looked at me tensely and with hostility, stating brusquely that she was quite capable of taking care of her child herself, and that she was not at all in agreement with this plan. She was the mother, and it was she who should deal with her child. Mr. F. added that the child welfare office had been notified; they would organize round-the-clock care for the infant at home. The patient's mother had also arrived to care for the child for a while.

*Patient History*

Mrs. F. is the younger of two children, with a brother 4 years older than she. She could tell us very little about her relationship with her mother, who, according to her, was "a difficult woman." Her father had suddenly "keeled over dead" when she was 10. Either she had forgotten most of her early childhood experiences, or she failed to report them. During our initial conversations, Mrs. F. treated me in a very reserved and dismissive way, stressing that she was not there voluntarily. Her answers were curt, or she remained silent while staring at the floor. She sketched out a fragmentary life story, characterizing it as "a normal life" without particular high or low points. She had gone to preschool and school, done professional training, married, and had a child. The patient neither expressed nor mentioned any affect along with the description of her life, but great affect was palpable in the countertransference and was overwhelmingly experienced by me as a tremendous diffuse tension. Only much later, when Mrs. F. was feeling better, did I learn that her mother "had sacrificed herself for her children and done everything for them." She had "ruled over" the home like a "mother hen"; she was always active and looking after the children. She had suffered from "depression," however, and had been admitted for inpatient treatment several times because, Mrs. F. said, "she wanted to take her life." The patient neither could nor would recall these times. She only remembered images of the emergency care physician, the police, the ambulance, and the psychiatric clinic.

These events occurred while Mrs. F was in elementary school. At about the same time, her father died unexpectedly of cardiovascular disease. Since then, her mother had constantly "leaned on her children for support, and clung to them." The thought that her mother was now taking care of her little daughter made Mrs. F. "completely crazy." For this reason, she pressed constantly to be discharged, and wasn't willing even to consider inpatient treatment. Initially she lacked insight into her illness; later on, she was unable to assess what she would be able to achieve in terms of her relationship with her infant. After each weekend pass her symptoms became worse, and she felt completely exhausted and overburdened.

### Consideration of Attachment Dynamics

Although the patient's history is fragmentary, it may be assumed that Mrs. F grew up with a very difficult relationship with her mother; this may be characterized as a disorganized/ambivalent attachment. Although the patient's mother seems not to have suffered any psychotic breaks with associated neglect or abuse, she had clearly suffered repeated bouts of illness, with depressive phases that included suicide attempts or suicidal thoughts that required inpatient treatment. We may suspect that Mrs. F experienced her relationship with her mother in childhood as very inconsistent, possibly even as "hot and cold," alternating between exaggerated or controlling overprotectiveness and the breaks in the relationship that resulted from the trauma of her mother's suicide attempts. During her depressive phases, Mrs. F's mother was undoubtedly not emotionally reachable, and she was probably also unreliable in her caregiving behavior and the sensitivity of her interactions. The patient would not have been able to experience her mother as a haven of safety and a secure base for exploration. Furthermore, during her mother's so-called healthy phases, the patient felt controlled, dominated, and confined in her ability to explore.

Mrs. F., now a mother herself who has to relate to her baby daughter, reacted with disorganized caregiving patterns similar to her own mother's; these were characterized by alternations between relational closeness and constancy toward the child, on the one hand, and disruptions in the relationship that were difficult for outsiders to comprehend, on the other. This interactional behavior was observed very early on. Mrs. F's attachment history, however, does not explain her fantasies, or the urge to kill her child. We may suspect that the depressive images contained in the fantasies were originally associated with her mother, then directed against her own inner child—her own self—and now projected onto her actual child. Attachment theory provides no adequate explanation for this painful process, which may be better described as an instance of projective identification: Mrs. F. learned as a child from her mother's rapidly changing and inconsistent behavior to control both the fear she felt as a result of her mother's encroachments and the fear (and aggression) that resulted from the relational disruptions, so as not to endanger further her relationship with her mother. These very early, and therefore now unconscious, fears and aggressions, arising out of mother–infant interaction patterns, had presumably been stored and suppressed in procedural memory. They were now reactivated in the relationship with Mrs. F's own child, where they burst out of the past and into the open. To an outsider, her symptoms appear to be psychotic fantasies because there is no immediately accessible understanding of the conflict. In fact, Mrs. F herself has neither memory of nor emotional access to her aggressive impulses, because the early interactional experiences and associated aggressive affects are stored only in procedural memory. Thus, her own unconscious aggression manifests itself in fantasies of killing her child, while at the same time she entertains unconscious fears that her mother could do something to *her* child.

It will be very important in the therapeutic process to establish an effective therapeutic safety net. The secure base offered to Mrs. F. in therapy must be sufficiently strong, sensitive, and predictable that it will be able to contain her emergent aggressive impulses.

*Therapy and Course*

During the first 3 weeks of treatment I spoke with Mrs. F. for 5 minutes three times a day. More prolonged contact was not possible, because of her intense defensiveness and her aggressive tension, and because of the clearly palpable mistrust that I experienced in the countertransference. Our interactions were precisely planned, scheduled, and firmly tied into the structure of the day. After a few days, our short meetings became very important to her; she sat expectantly by my door before each one. As time went on we became able to extend our conversations to two 10-minute sessions, then to two 20-minute sessions, and finally, toward the end, to one session of approximately 40 minutes daily. This process reminded me of the changes that take place in frequency and duration while breast-feeding a developing child.

In contrast to my usual technique of leaving the structure of therapy to the patient (particularly in cases of relationship–resistant attachment strategies), in this case my technical approach focused on providing a safe structure. In her ambivalence and insecurity, the patient was not left to think about the frequency of our meetings; rather, she found a therapeutic net of relational contacts and structures, the purpose of which was to give her a feeling of greater security. Similar structuring of contact was provided by the care personnel and by the structure of the unit itself. Trust developed in this patient not only as a result of the individual relationship with me, but over the entire course of treatment in a therapeutic milieu.

During the early phase of Mrs. F.'s treatment, she wished only to be with her child, and it was horrifying for her to think of the baby in the care of her own mother. However, we were able to come to an arrangement with her husband, whereby he would take over care of the infant during his vacations and whenever he was able to take time off from work. He would also bring the child with him to the unit as often as possible.

The patient began to take care of the infant with her husband; she could now also take long walks and visit home. In this respect, the husband was an important secure base, on whom Mrs. F. could rely without reservation. There had already been indications of this when she arrived for inpatient admission clinging to his hand. As she gained self-confidence and competence in caring for the infant, she was able to discuss with her husband that he might take more of a backseat and let her take over more of the caring for the child.

Mrs. F.'s impulse to kill the child receded increasingly into the background as a result of ongoing neuroleptic medication. It was very hard to discuss her murderous impulses with her, because as she became healthier she was deeply shocked and upset by them. The attachment history that presumably underlay her aggressive impulses was not accessible to conscious processing, so completely split off was it from the patient's experience. But as she became increasingly more competent in taking care of the baby, both on the unit and at home with her husband, there was no further reason not to discharge her from the clinic and set up outpatient treatment.

I was not involved in her further outpatient care, but I know that Mrs. F. continued to receive outpatient psychiatric and drug treatment.

*Concluding Remarks and Follow-Up*

This example points to a problem in Germany: in cases of early postpartum psychosis, mother and child are admitted to psychiatric clinics together only under exceptional circumstances. There is an urgent need that this be remedied in the future. In Germany (in contrast to Great Britain, for example) the consequence of postpartum psychotic illness is that the infant must be placed with family caregivers or with strangers, and eventually may have to be placed in foster care. The mothers lose contact with their children over the course of their inpatient treatment, and the result is emotional estrangement from the baby if nobody in her family can provide caregiving in the way Mrs. F.'s husband did. In Great

Britain both mother and child are admitted to the unit during the course of the mother's treatment, so that the mother and child do not have to be separated. It is almost always possible to help them form and maintain an attachment relationship, and they can usually continue to develop their relationship after the illness has subsided.

This example also illustrates how difficult, even impossible, it is to use an attachment-oriented approach in working through very early attachment relationships, which, like the aggressive affects in this case, are presumably stored in procedural memory. We are navigating through preverbal early childhood developments, and these experiences and affects are very difficult to access in verbal therapy. They seem to be processed best through an understanding of transference and countertransference, or by such nonverbal psychotherapeutic techniques as art, movement, or music therapy. This requires prolonged treatment. Nevertheless, attachment theory can provide an understanding of the early trauma of rapidly changing and inconsistent caregiving, as was the case with this patient, and it can give us the theoretical background to understand the need for a consistent, dependable relational structure within a clear and comprehensible therapeutic framework.

## The Trauma of Prematurity

Premature birth, especially extreme prematurity, is a traumatic experience for parents and can greatly impede the attachment process because of the infant's need for intensive care and prolonged confinement in an incubator. Earlier losses and separations can become reactivated in the mother's memory, and this can further hamper the establishment of attachment to the premature child (Brisch et al., 1996).

### Initial Presentation and Symptoms

I meet Mrs. L. in a consultation. The nurses in the pediatric intensive care unit notice that she is withdrawing increasingly from her extremely tiny newborn, who weighed slightly less than 2 pounds at birth. She had been highly involved with her child at first, visiting the unit at all hours, and calling the physician daily to inquire about the baby's progress. Now she visits more rarely, calls less often, and hardly ever wants to hold the infant. The nurses don't understand this behavior; the newborn's initially critical condition has stabilized, and the grave complications that Mrs. L. had feared have not set in.

Mrs. L. responds hesitantly to the offer of psychotherapeutic assistance, but she arrives punctually for our first appointment. We had agreed to meet at the incubator, where Mrs. L. proudly showed me her little daughter and, beaming with pleasure, informed me of all of her minor and major developments.

At this first meeting Mrs. L. immediately stresses that she understands why psychotherapy had been suggested. The nurses had talked with her about the fact that she had recently been visiting less. At first she hadn't noticed, but, now that she has looked at it more closely, she realizes that the nurses may well be correct. Somehow she feels more distant from the baby than she did immediately after her birth. She doesn't understand it herself, because she had been sitting by the incubator every day for 3 weeks, sometimes for many hours, thinking about and participating in the care of her daughter. Mrs. L. is able to reflect and talk about herself in a very complex and insightful way. She wants to know why something has changed inside her.

*Patient History*

Mrs. L. grew up in very sheltered and structured circumstances. She was the older of two daughters, her sister being 2½ years younger. She briefly described her early life as satisfactory. Even now she can count on her mother, who has come for an extended visit and who is running the household so that Mrs. L. can spend many hours with her baby at the incubator. There appear to be few conflicts here. However, when Mrs. L. begins to talk about her father, she begins to cry. He had died in an intensive care unit while she was still pregnant with this infant. She had so wanted him to see her daughter. He would have been a very proud grandfather. In tears, she reports the many hours she spent in the ICU, sitting by her father's bed. While he was in a coma, she noticed how difficult each breath was for him, and before he died he had been placed on a respirator, which she found to be "an unbearable torture."

She had always wanted to have children, and as she sat by her father's deathbed, she thought constantly about her pregnancy and his imminent death. Even though her child arrived prematurely, it still came too late.

## Consideration of Attachment Dynamics

Mrs. L. describes an early childhood of secure attachment. The way she has entered into the therapeutic relationship with me and her way of reflecting on her father's death and her experience of it both speak as well for security in her way of structuring relationships. It seems likely that she has not yet begun to process the death of her father and their long leave-taking in the intensive care unit. The grief process that is still taking place has overshadowed the necessary process of attachment to her premature infant, and this is all the more difficult in the context of the infant ICU and the incubator. It seems that the inpatient care of her premature child may remind Mrs. L. strongly of her father's death in intensive care, and of her own loss and grief.

## Therapy and Course

It was not hard for me to raise my suspicion that the necessary process of parental attachment to her child was being overridden by her grief over her father's death. Our conversations dealt intensely with the passing of her father, and her grief. The patient slowly became capable of greater emotional openness with her baby, expressed by more visits to the unit and her increasingly frequent wish to take her daughter out of the incubator and hold her. During this time she was also able to talk with her mother in the evenings about her relationship with her father. In this way, she could once again fall back on her mother as a secure base, both in conversation and in the current caregiving situation.

## Concluding Remarks and Follow-Up

Mrs. L. had no further serious difficulties strengthening her attachment relationship with her child, and this case should be seen as an example of crisis intervention from the point of view of attachment theory. It demonstrates how the necessary attachment process—in this case complicated by prematurity—can be overlain and disturbed by simultaneous separation and grieving processes as well as grief work. I suspect that without therapeutic assistance the formation of bonding with the premature child might have taken longer. Preoccupied with her grief, which had been reactivated by her experience in the infant ICU, Mrs. L. had not been able to open herself to her child optimally so that the necessary mother–child relationship could be established. In terms of usable resources, however, she was able to count on her mother as a secure base and find support in dealing with reality, working through her grief. This case demonstrates how existing positive attachment relationships can become activated and serve as "protective factors" in stressful situations. These should be promoted, thought through, and made use of in psychotherapy.

Even a secure attachment strategy does not protect one from dramatic and traumatic life events; however, it is a resource that can allow a person to better come to terms with such events, perhaps with the assistance of a therapist or other person.

~

## ATTACHMENT DISORDERS IN CHILDHOOD

Up until now, I have been describing maternal attachment disorders and their effect on the development of the mother's bond with the child. Now I will switch my focus to the development of pathological attachment patterns in young children. After having described maternal attachment disorders, it is easier to explain how attachment disorders of child and parent mesh in "statu nascendi." Moreover, the development of attachment disorders in children is easier to describe because children's life stories are shorter, and any traumatic events do not lie in the distant past.

For each of the forms of attachment disorder that I have already described in the overview in Section II ("Attachment Disorders"), I will present a separate case example.

## No Signs of Attachment Behavior

*Initial Presentation and Symptoms*

Five-year-old M. is brought in by his foster mother because of difficulties in preschool. Even after a year and a half in the program, M. has still made no friends. He prefers to play alone, both in preschool and at home, and withdraws completely for hours at a time. So, although she describes him as "easy to take care of," she has not been able to make emotional contact with him. He lives in a world of his own, in which he "hides as if behind a wall." He has never shown any signs that he misses her. She is worried about what this kind of behavior means for his future in school and in life. She and her husband would like to adopt the child, and they are still hoping that M.'s behavior will change and that he will show his foster parents that he is forming an attachment to them. At present, however, they are uncertain whether to adopt him—because he may well reject them—and they fear that perhaps they are not the right parents for him.

*Patient History*

M. was placed in his present foster family when he was 2 years old. He had been severely neglected, both physically and emotionally, during his first year in his family of origin. He spent his second year in a variety of foster care situations and in a pediatric clinic, where he was repeatedly admitted for short periods for neurodermatitis, bronchial infections, and possible asthma. By the time he was 2, he had spent a total of almost 12 months as an inpatient in pediatric clinics with only short breaks—malnourishment and neglect had been the reasons usually given for admissions during his first year. The rest of M.'s history is not well known. The mother was apparently an alcoholic who lived in a succession of relationships. The foster parents do not know whether M. has siblings. According to them, M. made himself at home in the family quickly and without problems. His contact with their 7-year-old son was good: there was "little fighting and friction, but not much playing together, either."

While his foster mother is telling his story, M. is playing in the room without visible emotional participation. We are able to talk undisturbed. As they get ready to leave, M. suddenly and unexpectedly clings to me and begins to cry because he wants to stay. His foster mother and I are both very surprised by this behavior. She explains it by saying that perhaps he has become fascinated by the new toys in my office. I note in the countertransference that I am very irritated by M.'s behavior; I would not have expected it, given his foster mother's description. At the same time, I don't really feel moved emotionally by the child's reaction; rather, his abrupt and immediately expressed closeness evokes in me more of a distancing reaction.

### Diagnostic Observations of Play

I observe M. over several play sessions to help me make a diagnosis before beginning treatment. The boy separates from his foster mother without problems and accompanies me into the playroom, with which he is already familiar. After a period of wandering around the room, he discovers a wooden train. He calmly and carefully puts together the wooden tracks; he makes them open at the ends, however, so that they do not form a continuous loop. M. places a number of small human figures on the train. During the trip they get in and out; some of them fall off and lie next to the tracks. The train derails each time, because the track ends—the train falls over, and all the remaining passengers spill out. M. then puts the train together with a great deal of intuitive feeling and attention to detail, and the game begins all over again. The train now runs in the opposite direction and derails at the other end. M. repeats this game several times, never saying a word to me. He makes no eye contact, seems immersed in his own world, and never comments on his play. However, from his nonverbal gestures and in the countertransference I recognize that he is extremely tense. After he allows the train to derail for the third time, I say, "Oh dear, the poor people! In *another* accident. Who's going to help them?" To this, M. has no visible reaction.

### Consideration of Attachment Dynamics

I suspect that with his very unstable family situation and his early neglect by his alcoholic mother, M. has been unable to develop a secure emotional attachment. Instead, he has undergone repeated, unpredictable separations and stays in the hospital, with changing foster care situations and new sets of caregivers. To an outside observer, as M.'s present foster mother reports, M. demonstrates no attachment behavior. His brief emotional reaction to me at the end of our first conversation speaks to this in an almost paradoxical way, because the separation reaction he demonstrated was to a stranger, something that his foster mother had apparently not observed previously. I suspect that M. might have a number of contradictory, incomplete, or fragmentary inner working models with respect to attachment. However, the most stable one appears to be to make himself unavailable to any attachment whatever, and withdraw completely into himself. This is the pattern that he lives out over the play sessions that I observed. His game with the train was perhaps the clearest demonstration of it, demonstrating at the symbolic level how M. continually "derails"—remains uncared for; there is nothing at the end of the track except another accident. Return trips follow the same pattern. Shuttled back and forth between a variety of potential attachment figures, M. presumably feels that he is continually falling out of incipient attachments, being given away, without adequate care during these separations. I suspect that this child has developed an emotional attachment to his current foster parents but that he cannot show it; his previous experiences lead him to fear that the old pattern of "falling off the train" might repeat with his new foster parents. The strongly symbolic quality of the train scenario moved me greatly, and made me hopeful that it would be possible to work with M. symbolically in play therapy. I interpreted his play as an indication of a spontaneous transference with hopes and desires for attachment; without such hopes he would not have expressed this symbolism in his unconscious play, which perhaps betrayed as well the hope of finding—in me in particular—a way out of the vicious cycle of repeated train accidents.

In this case, the problem of attachment is so strongly evident that conflicts relating to drive dynamics from the anal or oedipal period, as might be expected at his developmental age, are insignificant in comparison.

*Therapy and Course*

A 3-year course of twice- or thrice-weekly play therapy ensued, including regular, sometimes weekly, conversations with the foster parents.

The child's withdrawn play was the most important aspect of the initial phase of treatment. In the countertransference, feelings of emptiness and aloneness showed me that I was feeling unimportant, disregarded, and not even perceived.

Although M. preferred to play with concrete things like the train or building blocks, during the middle phase of treatment he switched to the sandbox. It was notable that at first he could not mold the sand. He finally spent a number of hours filling the sandbox with water, flooding it, as he himself was cathartically flooded by his own affects, which were under high internal pressure. It seemed to me that M. was affectively moved during this phase, and for the first time he was able to avail himself of offers of caregiving or assistance in structuring the situation, setting limits, and receiving support while he worked with the sand and water. I had some concern over the fact that this phase in the therapy, which from a classical perspective could be seen as a regression, would be followed by the 3-week break of my vacation.

When I joyfully greeted M. on my return, he dashed into my office and began to "greet" me with fists, kicks, and aggressive outcries. This reestablishment of contact, his rage at the pause in therapy, and the separation lasted a total of 20 minutes, during which time M. could barely be calmed. In the countertransference, I recognized his clear desire for closeness and physical contact with me, which he now expressed in aggressive form. It was very difficult for me to hold him physically, protecting myself from his blind rage and emotional violence, while at the same time keeping his desire for closeness in mind.

Without a background in attachment theory, I would have understood this outbreak as a Mahlerian "crisis of rapprochement" (Mahler et al., 1975), or from the Kleinian point of view as an expression of archaic destructive impulses (Klein, 1946). From the perspective of attachment theory, however, this behavior was clearly to be seen as a first reaction to separation, with both pronounced attachment behavior and anger at being abandoned. It may well be that in his protest M. was only showing the tip of the iceberg in terms of his early anger at separation, his aggression, and his disappointments about the many separations he had experienced. Presumably he had learned to suppress his feelings over time, because they did not prevent the separations occasioned by the child welfare office or his stays in the hospital.

Then followed a period during which M. acquiesced to separation from his foster mother at the beginning of each play session only under protest. I explained this clear attachment behavior with protest on separation (such as we often see in younger children) to his foster mother as a sign of progress. At the height of these separation outbursts and protests, she had to spend the entire play session with M.; later she spent only a short amount of time in the room with us. Occasionally M. would run out of the room during the session to make sure that she was still waiting for him. I myself was very relieved; I could see that his attachment behavior toward his foster mother and toward me was becoming healthier. But treatment was complicated by the fact that M. was no longer so easy to care for—I had to explain to the foster parents why in my view this actually represented progress. It seems that M. was demonstrating separation and protest behavior at the preschool door, which neither the foster mother nor the preschool teacher were able to understand.

Over the course of treatment it became possible to interpret M.'s behavior at the beginning and end of sessions and at weekend and vacation separations. My first attempts to address his grief and pain were met with his demand to "Shut your trap!" But it was becoming increasingly important for him, for example, to take toys from the playroom home with him over the weekend, some of which he would bring back to the next play session and some of which he would return only after a longer period of time.

There followed a phase of age-appropriate conflict processing, in which themes of aggression, acted out with battles and knights' castles, became significant. Oedipal themes also began to arise in his dealings with his foster mother. At the end of one session, M. found it important to show her his great castle-in-a-sandbox, with the powerful knights who had fought and killed me.

M.'s foster father had agreed to bring him to therapy once a week;

the foster father's inclusion in the structure of therapy facilitated M.'s identification with him, and resolution of the oedipal conflict was eventually possible. However, as always, periods of separation were points of contention. Aggressive reactions were evident for a long time after vacations; however, I had by now become attuned to and internally prepared for them. For this reason, my countertransference reactions were no longer as intense. Toward the end of his treatment, it even became possible to talk to M. about his fantasies, feelings, and pain *before* upcoming separations, with the result that his reactions after them became less intense. Finally, he began to take toys from the playroom with him on his own vacations, and explained to his parents that he absolutely had to bring them along. He had developed a secure internal working model of me and of his foster parents, who decided to adopt him. During the initial and middle phases of treatment, they had been very ambivalent about taking this step.

Termination of treatment was preceded by a long period of preparation. It was discussed with the parents as well as with M., who vacillated between the insistence that he wanted therapy to last for "always" and the incipient recognition that he no longer wanted to come to treatment sessions because he would rather be playing with his friends and brother. Over a lengthy and ambivalent transition phase, we were able to work through themes of separation, rapprochement, and saying good-bye during the play sessions, partly through direct verbalization and partly in symbolic play. Finally, with a lengthy vacation and his upcoming enrollment in school ahead of him, M. and I said good-bye. I continued follow-up conversations at 4-week intervals with the parents, in order to support them with M.'s further development.

### Concluding Remarks and Follow-Up

From his very difficult and traumatic early childhood, and in spite of presenting a lack of clear attachment behavior, M. had developed into a lively and well-adjusted schoolchild who had been able to develop secure emotional attachment relationships with his foster parents. When treatment began, the development of attachment was the most significant problem, after which both anal and oedipal themes could be worked through. Seen against another background—that is, not of attachment theory—his aggressive behavior in particular would have been interpreted differently, and a different technique would have been called for. I can imagine that therapists whose techniques are more in line with Melanie Klein's concepts would have interpreted and dealt with his aggressive behaviors and destructive fantasies more directly and openly.

To date, M. has integrated into school without great difficulties. He has built up contact with a number of students (his "friends"), and has consistently sought close contact with teachers who are especially important to him.

## Undifferentiated Attachment Behavior

### Social Promiscuity

*Initial Presentation and Symptoms*

Eight-year-old S. is brought to me by staff members of a residential school because, even after 2 years of treatment there she continues to demonstrate indiscriminate attachment behavior. She talks to strangers she meets at the institution, in school, and on the street completely indiscriminately, but with considerable social skill, and she gets involved with them in "pseudo-relationships." She signals to passersby whom she has never met before that she needs help, and then goes with them, thus placing herself repeatedly in danger of sexual abuse.

*Patient History*

S. had been picked up by the police as a "street child." By her own account, she had "fended for herself" for several months. Investigative work showed that she was a war orphan from an eastern European country, and she had been told many times in the course of carefully conducted conversations that her parents were dead, but she was convinced that her parents were still alive and held fast to this conviction. Little is known about her early history and development, as she herself was unable to disclose any specific information. According to her, she had several siblings, but she couldn't say exactly how old they were. It is not clear when, where, and under what circumstances she became separated from her parents, or whether she witnessed their deaths.

### Consideration of Attachment Dynamics

There was no way to know whether her indiscriminate relational behavior and her attachment disorder existed before her separation from her parents, before their death, or before the start of the war. The trauma of the loss of her parents, which she denied, left her having to fend for herself. She did this by seeking out relationships indiscriminately, that is, her disturbed behavior had an adaptive function and ensured her survival. The staff had expected that with continuous therapeutic guidance she would give up this pattern and open herself to specific attachment relationships with staff members at her residential school. Unfortunately, this had not occurred. One potential reason for this might be her refusal to grieve the loss of her parents and her persistent hope that she would find them again. Perhaps she was constantly seeking out sequential short-term relationships to see whether they might be her natural attachment figures. She might also have been protecting herself from the necessary grief work over her parents by creating short-term pseudo-attachments. Her failure to attach to the personnel at the residential school might mean that they were not sufficiently knowledgeable in attachment theory and were not working with the concept of attachment security.

### Therapy and Course

I did not treat this child myself, but supervised the staff members at the institution. It turned out that they had thought of S.'s behavior from a behavioral point of view. It was understandable that, in the short term, S. was continually reinforced in her behavior by a succession of ever-changing indiscriminate offers of relationship, which is why she saw no reason to change. Sanctions placed on her by the staff in the form of house arrest met with little success. But the perspective of attachment theory made clear that, while she repeatedly *began* to develop discriminating relationships with individual staff members, all of these efforts had been frustrated by the fact that several staff members had left the school. In spite of arranging a "system of support figures," it had not been possible for her to experience constancy of caregiving in the sense of a primary attachment over the past 2 years.

Once given a foundation in attachment theory, the staff came to understand how urgently necessary such constancy of relationship is for the formation of attachment security. The only way that S. could be expected to give up her indiscriminate relational behavior on the street would be if a secure base could first be successfully established with a staff member at the school. So far, she had felt like the "relationship orphan" there, and so it had made little sense for her to be open to a stable attachment relationship. Attachment theory provided a context in which contact between a female staff member and S. could be strengthened, and over the course of treatment an almost symbiotically close relationship developed between S. and this staff member. S. reacted to shift changes, free weekends, and vacations with vehement separation protest. Occasionally she ran away, and at those times she would again demonstrate her old attachment pattern on the street. As it eventually became evident that the necessary constancy of relationship had not been adequately provided over a long period of time, the decision was made to find a foster family for her. The institution and the youth welfare office discussed the girl's problems with the potential foster parents from the point of view of attachment theory.

The foster parents were able to take part in psychoeducational and therapeutic conversations with the staff. These focused on the importance of relationship constancy for establishing a secure attachment base. They learned about S.'s early history and the indiscriminate attachment behavior that resulted from it, which she used as a sort of defense, or coping mechanism. This preparation was necessary to keep the foster parents from feeling personally rejected or injured if S. were to run away or make friendly relationships with complete strangers.

After appropriate preparation, it was possible to place S. in a foster family. After about 6 months she began to show definite attachment behavior, with protest on separation and seeking closeness to her foster parents.

*Concluding Remarks and Follow-Up*

Consultation with the foster parents indicates that the undifferentiated attachment behavior that manifested itself in running away has completely disappeared, and that S. has developed a very stable attachment relationship to them.

Although S.'s behavior could be explained and understood from a learning theory perspective, the behavior modification techniques dictated by this perspective and initially used to treat S. had been largely unsuccessful. By focusing the staff's attention on the theoretical concept of a secure base, it was possible to change *their* perspective and behavior. Working together with the child welfare office also opened the possibility of placing S. in a stable home with foster parents where she would be able to develop an attachment relationship. However, if we had not provided the foster parents with the necessary information about attachment concepts and explanations of S.'s behaviors, even before the foster relationship began, their irritation at complications in the foster relationship might have appeared relatively early, which could have led them to terminate the foster relationship.

It is probable that S.'s indiscriminate attachment behavior served as a defense against the grief work required by the traumatic loss of her parents. For this reason, we recommended that the foster parents keep the possibility of therapeutic treatment for the child in mind because of her war trauma.

## Accident-Prone Behavior

*Previous History and Symptoms*

In 2 years 4-year-old F. has accumulated such a large file that the outpatient pediatric surgery staff is amazed by it. The boy is known to the doctors and nurses as a "regular customer," and when he is brought in by his parents with injuries—for the umpteenth time—they greet him accordingly. He comes in for accidents and injuries, not merely for such trivialities as abrasions, cuts, and lacerations. He has already needed inpatient care for craniocerebral trauma with concussion.

I am brought in as a consultant, and the outpatient physician tells me about the boy. He asks doubtfully about whether such behavior as in this situation can be considered normal, whether he should be concerned, and whether psychotherapy might be indicated. He has noticed that, even though the boy keeps coming back with injuries, he is always friendly and happy when he is brought in. This is quite a contrast with the behavior of other 4-year-olds who have been treated in the unit before. They remember it and kick and scream as soon as they reach the door.

*Patient History*

From a social history that my colleague had taken, I learn that both of F.'s parents are employed. Three children, aged 4, 8, and 12, are left at home unsupervised for many hours, cared for only by the 12-year-old. Even though F. shows no external signs of neglect, there are indications of emotional neglect. I remarked on the fact that F. preferred to engage in the fearless play that involved him in accidents during the evening, when both of his parents had come home from work exhausted; his behavior promptly engaged their attention and caregiving.

*Consideration of Attachment Dynamics*

My colleague knows nothing about F.'s early childhood development. However, the social history indicates clearly that he has not been cared for by his parents in a way that would support a secure attachment. His most secure relationship seems to be with his 12-year-old sister, who is responsible for him as the primary attachment figure. I suspect that although F.'s evening accidents ensure his parents' attention and caregiving on a behavior level, his internal motivation might be interpreted as seeking attachment to them. From a behavioral therapy perspective, F.'s behavior is maintained and reinforced by his parents' attention and the time-consuming and intensive treatment he receives in the outpatient unit. Not until the issue of attachment is considered can a deeper motivation for this behavior be appreciated. This view has consequences for treatment. It demands from the parents that they engage emotionally with their child, to form an attachment. They would have to spend more time with him and be more reliably available, and by so doing obviate the reason for the accidents. A behavioral approach, on the other hand, requires that the parents *not* react with attentiveness and caring to repeated accidents, and as the injuries require treatment, they are unlikely to be willing to do this. Furthermore, if we assume that the accident-prone behavior represents a deeper desire for attachment, ignoring it would probably increase accident frequency.

### Therapy and Course

No play therapy was undertaken with F.; his parents considered their son to be a "daredevil," and as they made clear to the physician and nurses during their next visit to the ambulatory unit, they were not able to understand attachment theory. It is rather doubtful whether attachment considerations would have any effect on these parents. On the other hand, the perspective and behavior of the outpatient personnel had changed. They no longer viewed F. merely as a child to be greeted in a friendly manner and then treated. They now felt more emotionally stricken when faced with F.'s behavior.

### Concluding Remarks and Follow-Up

Over time, it was noticed that F. and his parents came to the outpatient unit less frequently. Unfortunately, we do not know whether this was a result of changes in relational dynamics or simply because the parents now took their child somewhere else to be treated because of the confrontation that occurred in the outpatient unit.

Nevertheless, the perspective of the hospital personnel had been broadened by the view of this child's attachment dynamics, so that they now realize that frequent surgical needs in a child may conceal wishes and fears based on these dynamics.

## Exaggerated Attachment Behavior

### Excessive Clinging

#### Initial Presentation and Symptoms

The mother of 5-year-old P. calls pediatric psychiatry to make an appointment—not for the child, but for herself. The reason for her call is her son's refusal to go to preschool. P. urgently needs treatment, according to her, because, after all, he is going to start school when he is 6.

The mother arrives punctually at our scheduled meeting, holding P.'s hand firmly as she comes in. P. has refused to leave his anorak at the coat rack, and he sits on his mother's lap. He is a strong little blond boy with dark button eyes—a nice-looking child whose looks alone should make him a teacher's pet. His mother, barely 30, is very attractive. I notice later that she is somewhat overweight, which in fact she skillfully conceals by wearing an ample dark blue dress. With her widely draped dress and her son pressed close to her body, nestled in and seeming to shrink in her arms, she looks like a Madonna with child. I encourage P. to go over to the toy corner and look around and play with whatever he wants while his mother tells me some things. But P. glances over at the toys only briefly, and then presses even closer to his mother. She has made this appointment on the advice of a teacher, who considers P.'s behavior unusual for his age, and the parents are concerned about how P. will manage school next year if he doesn't even want to go to preschool alone. His mother reports attempts to separate at the preschool door that end in panicked screaming. "With a heavy heart," she says, she then takes him back home. In addition, P. has no friends; he plays only at home, preferably with his mother.

*Patient History*

The mother reports that P. is her first and only child. The pregnancy was "the most beautiful time" of her entire life—only the actual birth did she remember as "terrible." Shortly after it she was ill for a time; this on questioning turned out to be an episode of postpartum psychosis, which resolved after 4 weeks of medical treatment. I learned nothing about the content of the psychosis, and it was clear that the mother didn't want to talk about it. She described the rest of P.'s childhood and development as typical and ideal. She felt that the lack of a stubborn phase was "healthy" and in no way peculiar, because she "can't stand stubborn children." Since P. couldn't nurse as a result of her illness, she continues to this day to make liberal use of a baby bottle when he goes to sleep, so that he can catch up on the nursing he missed.

Further questioning brought out other separation problems, at bedtime, for instance. P. could not go to sleep without his father or mother nearby. Usually he went to sleep in their presence on the sofa in the living room, with a baby bottle.

The father is very dedicated to his work and comes home late. P. is often allowed to stay up late in the evening so that he and his father can play together for a while. His mother has read that fathers are very important in boys' development. Because P. falls asleep late and she allows him to sleep in the morning, she cannot get him to preschool as early as the teachers expect.

The mother then jumped up suddenly, put the frightened P. on the floor, and without a word of explanation ran out of the room. I was completely nonplussed by this behavior. P. was crying and screaming shrilly, but he did not follow his mother. I tried to calm him by sitting on the floor next to him and suggesting that we play a game with a toy car. I assured him that his mother would soon come back, and that I was there, too. However, I was irritated and alarmed about what was going on with his mother. After about 3 minutes, she returned—pleased with herself, but a little out of breath. She had forgotten to switch off the light in her car. With this explanation, she sat down on the chair again and placed P. on her lap without further comment, although he had just begun to get interested in a police car. P. seemed to let everything wash over him, but this time he did not nestle as he had earlier. He sat up straight on his mother's knees and began for the first time to explore the playroom with curious eyes.

I handed him the police car, and P. began to play with it on the table. He whined and cried continuously as he played; in part this seemed to indicate that he wanted help, and in part it seemed like attention-getting. Finally, he made a show of throwing the car onto the floor and then snuggling up to his mother. After some hesitation, he accepted my renewed offer of the car, and he resumed his play with it on the table. His mother spoke words of attempted comfort, telling him that he "shouldn't act so silly." At the same time, she turned her attention to me and commented, "Now you have seen it 'live.' P. won't let me out of his sight, and when I leave for even a moment, he creates a terrible stir."

I used this scene to talk to her about my irritation at her disappearance; I had been concerned. She was surprised that it had made any difference to me, as it had only been for a moment. She reported that she left P. at the preschool door quickly—otherwise, she wouldn't be able to get away.

I suggested to her that P. might have had the same reaction that I had just now when she left him without a clear good-bye at the preschool door. This was a completely new idea to her, because up to now she had always disappeared quickly in hopes that P. wouldn't notice; she wanted to get away before he started screaming, something that she couldn't bear.

*Consideration of Attachment Dynamics*

Presumably, P.'s early infancy had been disturbed as a result of his mother's difficulties with separation at the end of her pregnancy and her psychotic episode. The scene in my office during our initial conversation was an indication that the mother clings to P., leaving him little room for exploration, while at the same time separating herself from him abruptly out of her own problems with separation, as during our initial conversation and at the preschool door. P.'s excessive clinging was in the foreground of the picture, while the aggressive behavior seen in the ambivalent insecure pattern of attachment was less evident. However, the mother's difficulties with separation, as well as her insensitivity in caregiving and in interaction, clearly form the backdrop for this attachment disorder. Nevertheless, my interactions with P. suggest possibilities for interesting him in exploration and helping him to get over the school separation. I am reminded of his relationship with his father, who, in spite of his professional involvement, finds time to play with his son in the evening. P.'s excessive clinging, along with a massive attachment disorder, leads to pronounced problems with separation accompanied by very inhibited exploration. This is demonstrated not only at the preschool door but also at bedtime, when the 5-year-old can't fall asleep in the absence of his parents.

*Therapy and Course*

I recommended play therapy for P., but this was unimaginable to the mother because, in her opinion, P. could not separate from her for so

long. The father saw things differently, but the mother's categorical
"No" frustrated this plan. She wanted "parental counseling," the goal of
which would be that her child would be able to enter preschool and
eventually school. Treatment therefore consisted of once a week "counseling" (actually therapy for the mother) and sessions that included the
father about every 3 weeks. The mother liked this arrangement. She
wanted more frequent contact, which she arranged between sessions by
telephone, with questions about P.'s behavior and about what she
should do.

The difficulty P.'s mother experienced with separation from her
child took center stage in this work. She herself had a very close, almost
symbiotic, relationship with her own mother, with whom she spoke on
the phone several times a day. She felt very insecure about her own parental competence, and she had marked problems with self-esteem that
extended beyond child-rearing. Increasingly over the course of therapy,
I became the mother's secure base. As a result of this, after 3 months she
became able to take her son to preschool in the morning and manage
the separation with the help of the teacher, knowing that immediately
afterward she would come to me for her session. The therapy arrangements helped her feel sufficiently safe that she could separate from her
son in the morning. Over the course of the therapy, I was able to speak
with the father and to conclude that he was behaving increasingly as a
supportive attachment figure. As often as possible, he planned his business activities in such a way that he would be the one to take his son to
preschool. A telephone call from the teacher made it clear to me that
she was trying to help P. deal with the separation by involving him in
play with other children as quickly as possible on his arrival. I asked her
to consider that P. would first have to develop a secure foundation with
her before he would be able to use her as a secondary attachment figure
despite his ambivalent attachment to his mother. This intervention, and
a new arrangement at the preschool, with time set aside in the morning
for individual care from the teacher, made it possible for the boy to become more independent and separate from his mother with little protest.

After about 6 months, P. was able to go to preschool in the morning
as a matter of course, and the parents considered that the goal of

therapy had been achieved. The mother felt that there was no further reason for therapy, especially since the boy's bedtime behavior had also changed. He was now able to go to sleep in his own bed if the door was open and the light was on. It was important to P. that his father take him to bed.

*Concluding Remarks and Follow-Up*

Undoubtedly, this treatment was only a temporary solution to an acute problem. The mother's pronounced problems would have required lengthier therapy, and she mentioned this possibility at our final session. Whether or not she will make use of it remains an open question. P.'s father's involvement played a considerable role in the success of therapy and in P.'s changed behavior. He made separation easier for his son while at the same time introducing him to the world of exploration. The behavior of the teacher was just as important. She took care of P. after the morning separations from his mother by offering him short periods of individual attention, thereby giving him the opportunity to establish a secure base with her as secondary attachment figure.

My relationship with the mother may have functioned as a secure base, making the morning separations from her son easier to handle, especially on days when the therapy sessions occurred immediately after she took her son to preschool. I doubted the stability of this "successful therapy," however, and told the parents that they should feel free to call me at any time if separation problems recurred or if there were other difficulties. I later learned from the father that P. had developed "quite well," and that he had been proud about entering first grade.

## Inhibited Attachment Behavior

*Initial Presentation and Symptoms*

I am called in to consult on the peculiar behavior of a 3-year-old girl. N. has been admitted for planned surgery. The nurses have noted that N. appears timid and overly compliant, in that she was highly cooperative and underwent all examinations and preoperative procedures "without crying or whining." One look from her mother was enough to make N.

overcome her hesitation when blood was being drawn. She showed no clear separation reaction when her mother left. The pediatric nurses reported that, as soon as her mother left, the girl, who had previously been so timid, became talkative and very active; she explored the unit and seemed to become a different person emotionally. They suspected that coercion might play a role in N.'s relationship with her mother.

*Patient History*

In my first conversation with the mother, who gives information readily, I learn that her pregnancy was normal and so was N.'s early development. N. has a 1-year-old brother, with whom she plays cooperatively. The mother has "no problems" with either child: "Both turned out well and do what I tell them." N. recently started preschool, which she really looks forward to. The mother knows of no separation problems. When they went out in the evening, they could leave N. alone with a babysitter, even when she was very young. I bring up the topic of N.'s peculiar behavior on admission. N.'s mother cannot understand our concerns about this "normal behavior of a normal child." According to her, N. had simply needed time to get used to the new situation; she is always very lively, and in preschool she is known to be a curious little girl. In response to my questions, the mother adds that she is very strict with N. at home, as you have to "make clear who makes the rules." Obedience is very important to her; a glance should be sufficient. Although she is prepared to mete out physical punishment, this has not been necessary because N. knows that she is serious. The threat of punishment alone suffices.

*Consideration of Attachment Dynamics*

I presume that N.'s peculiar and overly conforming behavior is an expression of her attachment relationship with her mother, which requires that she move within clearly set boundaries enforced by threats of punishment. These delimit both her attachment and her exploratory behavior. Inpatient admission and procedures such as blood-drawing must have been frightening to her, but she did not dare to show the expected comfort-seeking reactions to her mother out of fear of being punished for disobedience. She suppressed her attachment needs while her mother was present. I understand this excessive conformity to be a disorder, since the suppression of attachment needs in situations of fear can lead to elevated physiological reactions with somatic and psychosomatic consequences, similar to those found in avoidantly attached children.

*Therapy and Course*

No therapeutic bond could be established with N.'s mother. We had three more conversations during the time that N. was in the hospital, but my attempts to acquaint the mother with the implications of attachment theory went nowhere. She insisted that she had been brought up in the same way, and she expected her child to learn order, and right from wrong. She considered it progress that, although she herself had received many beatings as a child for disobedience, she was managing to raise her children by strictness alone.

*Concluding Remarks*

No follow-up information is available. However, this case illustrates why it is advisable to look for problems of attachment dynamics in children and adolescents whose behavior is overly conforming, especially when fear-provoking situations do not evoke age-appropriate expectable attachment behavior. Whether this situation causes psychosomatic disturbances related to stress and its elevated physiological reactivity is the subject of continued research.

## Aggressive Attachment Behavior

*Initial Presentation and Symptoms*

V., a 9-year-old schoolgirl, comes to me at the insistence of the child welfare office after she had physically attacked and injured her mother several times. Aggressive quarrels between daughter and parents were known to occur, and V. had already been suspended from school because of constant aggressive behavior toward other students.

Both parents arrive at our initial appointment drunk. Their 9-year-old daughter is with them, and they are accompanied by a caseworker. I am barely able to extract a structured history, because the parents feel like they are in a court of law. Summoned to appear by the child welfare office, they are boycotting the proceedings by remaining more or less silent. V. responds to my attempts at conversation with aggressive and provocative insults. She sizes me up exactly, tests my reactions, and swears at me repeatedly. When I discuss with her parents the possibility of inpatient treatment, V. begins to cry, clings to her mother, and protests that under no circumstances will she permit herself to be separated from her: "We stick together." A few minutes later she is heaping loud abuse on her mother, on the grounds that it is her fault if she, V., has to go into the hospital.

### Consideration of Attachment Dynamics

V. is the sixth child of her parents, who have been alcoholics for many years. She had very unstable early childhood relationships with both of them. The family has been known to the child welfare office as a "problem family" for a long time. V.'s older siblings (three children are in foster situations, and one sister lives in a home; only V. and the brother, who is 2 years older, live at home) have also had trouble with antisocial and aggressive behavior. Reports from the child welfare office make clear that aggressive quarrels with each other and with their children characterize the parents' day-to-day relationship style, especially when they are drunk. Presumably V. learned very early that aggression—primarily verbal aggression in the form of insults and provocation—are everyday forms of establishing attachment and contact. I experienced this very directly in our initial contact, as I saw V.'s insults as a way to create the possibility of a direct personal relationship with me. In her daily relationships with teachers and classmates, however, these aggressive ways of initiating relationships lead to the opposite result, as they are not understood to represent a desire for attachment and relationship. V.'s actions cannot be adequately explained at a purely behavioral level, because while her aggressive and insulting behavior does gain attention for her, it also ends up getting her rejected. From that perspective, continuing aggression makes no sense. From the point of view of attachment dynamics, however, V.'s aggressive behavior may be understood as an attachment disorder, a pattern of relating established in the course of aggressive quarrels with the mother. When the possibility of a separation (inpatient treatment) comes up, V. reacts with clear separation protests and plainly demonstrates that she is attached to her mother, though her attachment behavior is accompanied by the use of insults. Of course, these aggressive quarrels could also be an expression of rage and disappointment. However, in that case we would expect that she would set boundaries more clearly and distance herself from her mother, with whom she has a history of frustrating interactions with reason to believe that these frustrations will continue. Attachment theory makes it possible to understand the attachment of victims of abuse, coercion, and brutalization to the perpetrators.[4] For V., aggression is a familiar means of establishing and intensifying an albeit insecure attachment between herself and her mother.

*Therapy and Course*

It became evident over a few meetings that V.'s parents possessed neither the motivation nor the insight for psychotherapy. Yet, admission for inpatient treatment, while therapeutically sensible, nevertheless seemed unpromising because the experience with children like V. is that they soon run away from inpatient facilities and return home. Such behavior frustrates many institutions to the point where they are no longer prepared to cooperate, and these children may lead a "vagabond" existence, shuttling among the institutions to which they have been remanded, a variety of youth home and foster care situations, and their natural parents, with whom they seek out frequent periods of intense contact. In cases of abuse and maltreatment, parents in such family constellations often pull out all stops to discover the undisclosed places where their children are living.

We discussed with V., her parents, and the child welfare office the possibility of a group home for girls close to the family's neighborhood. Parents and child both agreed to this solution, and V. moved into the group home on a trial basis. This way the potential for attachment contact between V. and her parents was not precluded; instead, such contact could be cultivated under more structured conditions. The possibility of structured parental visits and weekend passes was considered and justified from the perspective of attachment theory in discussions with the staff of the group home.

Earlier in my career I would not have considered such an approach very promising and would have made a case for stricter separation from the parents and for inpatient child psychiatric care; I would not have proceeded from an assumption of attachment between parents and child, given their prior history of frequent aggressive quarreling. Given V.'s rage and disappointment, and her aggressive behavior toward her parents, I would have expected her to feel relief only if she were separated from them and not subject to further frustration.

### Concluding Remarks and Follow-Up

With her admission to a group home and with parental visits that maintained the relationship, V.'s development became calmer. She was able to attend school regularly again, and as her attachment to the caregivers in the home increased she became able to cultivate the relationship with her parents, taking into account her need for closeness as well as for distance—she learned to distance herself when her parents' drinking made them unavailable or when the aggressive quarrels arose, and fall back on helpful relationships in the group home. She no longer had to provoke her parents aggressively in order to achieve or maintain an attachment relationship with them.

In summary, I want to stress that attachment phenomena must be taken into account in cases of aggression, abuse, or brutalization. In general, we assume that it is necessary to separate the perpetrator and the victim. Unfortunately, there is as yet very little research on the effects that trauma has on attachment, on the one hand, and on the other, how separation conditioned by the trauma affects the development of children. Therapeutic approaches that allow for the possibility of physical separation with intermittent interaction in the form of structured visits between maltreating parents and child victims have, in my opinion, not been adequately tested because the theoretical principles involving attachment in the perpetrator–victim relationship have not been sufficiently considered and researched.

## Attachment Behavior with Role Reversal

*Initial Presentation and Symptoms*

Five-year-old D. is brought in to see me by her mother, who says that the child has refused to go to preschool for the past 3 months. The mother is not able to explain this behavior, as D. had always liked preschool.

Throughout our first conversation, D. maintains physical contact with her mother: she stands next to her, holds her hand, and looks directly into her mother's face. When the mother, describing the situation, begins to cry, D. climbs onto her lap, dries her tears with her hands, and comforts her mother by touching her tenderly.

*Patient History*

D. is her parents' only child, and the couple has recently separated. It came as a complete surprise to the mother when the father moved out and, as she says tearfully, her world "collapsed." According to her, D. had a very intimate relationship with her father; current visitation guidelines state that she is to visit her father every 2 weeks. The mother is very depressed about the separation and is receiving psychiatric treatment for depression. She believes that D. is suffering greatly by being pulled back and forth between her mother and her father. After visiting her father over the weekend, she is always "completely destroyed and disturbed." On Mondays, she is unable to separate from her mother and go to preschool.

During our second session the mother tells me that she threatened to kill herself and her daughter 4 months ago. D. was very upset about this and since then has not slept in her own bed, but in her father's former bed, next to her mother's bed.

The mother says that D. was an eagerly awaited child; she describes D.'s early development as unremarkable and ideal. She herself gave up her profession to devote herself to her family. D. had always been a lively and sunny child, curious and open. She loved preschool, and everyone there liked her. Now she is sad; she sits around, won't go to preschool, and doesn't even leave the house anymore. The father is to blame for everything because, in the mother's view, he abandoned the family.

### Consideration of Attachment Dynamics

I suspect that D. had a very secure attachment to her mother, but that the acute stress of her parents' separation has resulted in an attachment disorder with role reversal. D. experiences her mother as depressed. The mother is presumably clinging to her daughter since her separation from her husband, using her as an "attachment-antidepressant." Her threat to kill herself and her child has frightened D. considerably, so that she now worries even more about her mother. I observed this role reversal when D. comforted her mother in her grief, taking over a mother's responsibility. D. cannot continue her own normal exploratory behavior—going to preschool, getting together with friends—because of the vigilance demanded of her in her effort to support her mother. Over the weekends, when she is connected with her father and separated from her mother, she fears that the mother might kill herself in her depression. For this reason, the weekend visits represent a great attachment conflict. Attachment conflicts are typically found in children of divorced parents when attachment behavior and relationships with both parents exist, but here the situation is dramatically heightened because D. is not merely faced with a possible deterioration in the relationship with her mother if she turns to her father, but instead with the actual loss of her mother as a result of her depression and suicide threats.

### Therapy and Course

D.'s mother was willing to let D. begin play therapy, but she was skeptical about how it could improve D.'s behavior. Shortly after the initial consultation I received a call from the mother's attorney, asking me to provide an expert opinion, stating that D.'s emotional development was threatened by the weekend visits with her father. The mother had reported to the lawyer how very "disturbed" D. was after these visits.

Therefore, as the legal representative of his client, he was concerned for the well-being of the child. I attempted to explain that, although I was quite prepared to make myself available for treatment, I could not simultaneously act as an expert witness in a divorce proceeding. However, the mother and her attorney insisted on an expert opinion. Because I refused, our relationship ended, and there was no treatment.

*Concluding Remarks and Follow-Up*

This example makes clear how especially great is the role played by attachment dynamics in cases of separation or divorce, and how children may be plunged into conflicting attachment loyalties and ambivalent feelings about both parents. The expressed wish of many children that their parents should "get together again" is evidence of their efforts to resolve their attachment ambivalence. It is necessary to take these aspects of attachment dynamics into consideration with great therapeutic sensitivity both in the treatment of children and in discussions with their parents, so that the children, who are intensely attached to both parents, can maintain these attachments and find a new modus vivendi. If divorcing parents use or abuse their children's attachment capacities, needs, and relationships in order to resolve their own psychic conflicts (in this case a depressive suicidal crisis), then the typical attachment behavior characteristic of role reversal may occur. The children are expected to provide a secure attachment base for their depressed, injured, and suffering parents. They must satisfy their parents' attachment needs and stabilize them while suppressing their own fear of loss of the parents. It is important to realize that without therapeutic help a new pathological attachment may develop out of such paradoxical attachment relationships, which the children may then bring into later attachment relationships.

## Psychosomatic Symptoms

### Failure to Thrive

M. was referred to me by a pediatrician versed in endocrinology who has diagnosed failure to thrive. No hormonal cause could be determined, and he wondered whether the cause might be psychogenic.

*Initial Presentation and Symptoms*

M., a 14-month-old male infant, is brought to the initial consultation by his young parents (mother, 22; father, 25). The mother reports that during a recent medical checkup normal growth was found to have ceased, and repeated examinations confirmed that growth had in fact slowed. Tests to rule out hormonal disturbances found no pathology. Nevertheless, the mother is convinced that there are still tests that have not been done and that it is only a matter of time until some illness is found. She is very alarmed and cannot understand why she has been referred to a child psychotherapist. I experience both parents as distanced, dismissive, and reproachful. In the countertransference I sense clear rejection. They feel that they have been mandated to see me, misunderstood, and placed on the "psycho-track." With great patience I listen to the litany of detailed reports about tests already conducted and results obtained. The parents have also brought letters from a variety of physicians for my information. My impression is that these letters are meant to convince me of the organic genesis of the growth retardation.

M. is the first child of these parents. Four months ago the mother has begun working again; the father is professionally independent. He is very successful, apparently the result of his great dedication to his work—"he works day and night," his wife says. M. has been in family day care since his mother returned to work 4 months ago. She brings him in at 7:00 in the morning and picks him up again at 6:00. The daycare mother is very flexible and generous; the child occasionally sleeps over with her as well. M. is one of four children being cared for by this woman. Although M.'s mother sometimes gets the feeling that the day care mother is caring for the children "for profit alone," she is nonetheless pleased with her flexibility, because it allows her to work full-time in her old position. During our conversation, her son is sitting on the floor in a baby chair next to her. After a while he begins to whine and then becomes irritated. His mother manages to distract and quiet him by pulling a succession of toys out of her bag as if by magic. He plays with these for a while, but then throws them down and begins to whine again. I have the impression that M. wants to be taken out of his chair and into his mother's arms so that he can move, or perhaps even explore the playroom a little. I offer this possibility to the parents, but they both reject it on the grounds that M. would only want to be taken by the hand and led around the room, and then we wouldn't be able to talk anymore. The conversation finally ends when M. starts to cry, and the parents get up and terminate the conversation. The parents are prepared to come again "if we absolutely have to," but they don't see the point in it.

### Consideration of Attachment Dynamics

M. was a planned child of this young couple, both of whom are very dedicated to their jobs. My initial impression, confirmed by our later conversations, is that both parents demonstrate a rather aloof caregiving pattern; they respond in a functional and monotone way to their child's attachment and exploration needs. They interact with their child based upon their own needs. I suggest that they try to attune themselves sensitively to the child's signals and needs, but the parents neither accept nor act upon this advice.

In our first conversations I see reason to suspect a psychogenic causation of the retarded growth; an avoidant attachment disorder between parents and child may have led to emotional deprivation made even worse by the daycare situation. There M. is the fourth of four children, and, although he is physically well cared for, I suspect that the experience of emotional attachment that he needs is not sufficiently available, either from the daycare mother or from his parents. M. demonstrated clear attachment signals and sought closeness, but his parents neither understood these signals nor responded adequately to them. They felt that they risked spoiling him if they responded to his whining and took him out of his baby seat. "We want him to know what's what right from the start."

### Therapy and Course

As prescribed, the parents came every 2 weeks to sessions that took on the character of parent training. We talked about M.'s development, his wishes, needs, play, curiosity, and interests, and over time the parents became more adept at perceiving their child's signals and needs. A pediatrician, whom the parents viewed as their primary consultant, was seeing the child at the same time. As several weeks passed, the parents began to trust me more and to turn to me for answers to specific child-rearing questions. As a result, I was able to videotape a mother–child play interaction and to watch the video with the parents. They responded positively to this approach, which resembled the sensitivity training we had first used for interactional training with the parents of premature infants. Together we observed the child's behavior and reactions, his mother's responses to them, and the perceptions to which she gave priority. We also discussed other possible ways to respond. As a result, the parents' creativity increased, and it became easier for them to tune in to the child's inner world. (It is crucial when beginning this type of perception and sensitivity training to reinforce the parents' positive perceptions and behaviors so that they do not come to doubt their own competence, even when, as with these parents, competence at first seems to be in short supply.) After 6 months, M.'s growth curve began to normalize. He was now able to get about freely, and his parents could perceive his need for exploration—one of the things we discussed was how to make an apartment safe for a curious 2-year-old.

The parents and I continued to meet irregularly over the next 2 years. M.'s retarded growth, the presenting complaint, was no longer an issue because by then it had begun to normalize. The parents now came to me with questions about child development, and they made every effort "to do everything right." M.'s stubbornness, and the parents' original fear that they might spoil him, became the most important themes in therapy.

### Concluding Remarks and Follow-Up

The initial disorder, with its tendencies toward the development of emotional deprivation, was reversed in therapy. At no time during this period was M. treated with hormones, as no growth hormone deficiency was ever found. The parents' aloof caregiving and their low sensitivity to the child's signals improved over the course of their consultation and sensitivity training with me. This enabled them to interact with him more responsively and take better account of his age-appropriate need for exploration. It remains an open question whether and how their underlying dismissing attachment strategies were changed by these new experiences. Nevertheless, the child's attachment security appears to have been supported by the parents' changed interactional style in that the development of an extreme attachment disorder with psychosomatic reaction was avoided.

### Eating Disorders

*Initial Presentation and Symptoms*

A female friend of G.'s mother (whose own child I had once treated) calls to set up an appointment for her, asking whether I treat children with eating disorders. She accompanies her friend and her 8-month-old son, G., to the initial session.

At first glance, G. appears to be a normally nourished boy. He sits in his baby chair looking about curiously while his distraught mother reports that he is a poor eater and that she spends hours each day trying to feed him. Often her eyes fill with tears at his refusal to eat. Every week she visits the pediatrician, who weighs G. and gives her the same report: "No weight gain." All the tests for organic causes have come back negative, but she is convinced that something is wrong with her child, and further tests are scheduled. In the meantime she is at the end of her rope, and she dreads each next feeding. She is preoccupied with food. Finally, her friend suggested that she make an appointment with me; perhaps it is she who needs help more than the child. In fact, the mother is completely exhausted and despondent, and she begins to cry. While this is going on, G. is becoming increasingly agitated in his baby chair, and he wants to be held. She picks him up, but he continues to be agitated. The mother is not able to respond to him because she is preoccupied by her own thoughts and her narrative.

*Patient History*

G.'s mother is 25 years old, and G. is her first child. She reports that she and her husband had wanted a child. The pregnancy was apparently completely normal, although she tended throughout to brood and fret

about all the things that could possibly go wrong. She discussed pregnancy and birthing for hours on end with her mother and other women;
at times she got herself worked up at the thought that G. might be
handicapped, or even die at birth. When he had to be admitted to the
infant clinic for several days because of jaundice, it was enough to cause
her world to collapse. He was breast-fed for only a short time; she
apparently nursed him for only 3 weeks. It may be that lactation was
disturbed by her being upset. G. bottle-fed eagerly, but he often vomited
afterward. She was very worried about this and went to the pediatrician
for advice. When he established that G. was gaining weight slowly, she
went into a panic. She had been besieged with advice from all sides (especially from her mother) about how to feed G. She said that her
mother called almost every day to inquire about G.'s condition, always
wanting to know whether she had cooked meals and whether she herself was eating enough. Her mother was thus becoming involved with
all aspects of the household. G.'s mother feels that she is being watched
and controlled from all sides: by the pediatrician, by her mother, and
now perhaps by me as well. Her husband tries to support and relieve
her, but he works shifts and so a regular feeding schedule is not possible
long-term.

### Consideration of Attachment Dynamics

I suspect that the attachment of G.'s mother to her own mother is rather
ambivalent; her feeling of insecurity and of being controlled and
watched is consistent with this. In her distress, she calls her mother
often, but at the same time she wants to be able to care for and make decisions about her child on her own. Fears during pregnancy that the
child might be handicapped are not unusual. Apparently though, they
have taken on greater significance in this case because, in her fear and
distress, G.'s mother turns to many people, including her own mother.
However, she derives little security from doing so. Although the baby is
of normal weight, and there is no acute danger that he could starve, a
vicious cycle has developed. Because of her own insecurity, this mother
suffers from low self-esteem with regard to her maternal competence.
She spends hours with the child, completely fixated on feeding, while at

the same time she is extremely angry and irritated about this form of relationship. Because this is "a life-and-death matter," she naturally doesn't want to let her baby starve, and as a result is unable to set clear boundaries. She re-creates an ambivalent attachment pattern with her child, and feeding becomes the focal point of the ambivalent interaction. As a result, G. is actually developing an eating disorder with vomiting and refusal to eat.

*Therapy and Course*

I assured the mother that I did not want to be another person telling her what to do, but that I wanted to offer her support and safety in this difficult situation so that she herself would be able to determine when and how often to feed the child. Furthermore, I let her know that I could see quite clearly that she has a very loving relationship with her son. She has been made very unsure of herself by an overabundance of recommendations and second-guessing, especially from her own mother. She sighed loudly and agreed with me. We talked about whether it would help if I discussed with her pediatrician the possibility of not having G. weighed weekly, and letting her decide when to make an appointment for a weighing. At first the mother was relieved by this idea, but then she later added the caveat that she didn't want to deal with long waiting periods between calls and appointments; if she needed an appointment, the pediatrician would have to see her on short notice.

She also agreed with my suggestion that she call me whenever she felt the need, and I agreed to return her calls as soon as I could. At first she wanted to call before and after each feeding because she felt so tense, believing that each feeding "could only go wrong." For the first few days she made heavy use of the phone, and I was able to reassure her about the feedings. She convinced herself that everything would go well and that she would give G. the proper amount of food or, at my suggestion, allow her child to decide how much to eat. After each feeding I had to reassure her that G. would not starve, even if he took small portions, and that she did not have to justify this to her mother. Within a few days the interaction around feeding became less tense, and she felt calmed by our telephone conversations.

Her boundaries with her own mother became the focus of subsequent sessions. G.'s mother still wanted closeness and support from her own mother; at the same time she wanted to establish boundaries, and to assume primary responsibility for caring for and raising her child. Her entanglement in the relationship to her own mother, however, made it difficult for her to serve as a secure base for her own child. The relationship between G. and his mother was well on its way to an entrenched ambivalent attachment pattern, by way of an eating disorder, but, little by little, she was able to take steps toward establishing boundaries with her own mother, among other things by limiting their telephone calls to a single conversation per week. I suspect that this was possible because she could call me at will, using me as a secure base in therapy. Her contact with the pediatrician also became less tense because she no longer viewed him as a supervisor and because she could now regulate distance in accordance with her need for security and attachment.

Treatment stretched out over a total of 4 months, after which the eating disorder was less of a problem. However, we continued to meet at greater intervals every 2–3 weeks to discuss her interaction with her own mother as well as her son's increasing desire for exploration. At each session I allowed the mother to determine when our next meeting would be. This was followed by periods during which I saw her increasingly less often, a trend occasionally interrupted by upset telephone calls when she was "swamped" by the child's "incessant exploration."

### Concluding Remarks and Follow-Up

This case demonstrates how a woman's preoccupied "state of mind" with respect to attachment can be reproduced in her interaction with her own child and can crystallize symptomatically around an eating disorder. The particular symptom itself is undoubtedly variable; a similar pattern could arise in relation to sleep disorders, for example. Given her ambivalent attachment relationship with her mother, the emotional security that the mother receives in the therapy relationship allows her to be more relaxed in her interaction with her child and to work on the ambivalence in the relationship with her own mother. The possibility of her determining, herself, the frequency of sessions as well as the degree of closeness and distance with the therapist was helpful here.

From a classical psychodynamic perspective, it could be said that both the detachment from her own mother as well as a relaxation of the ambivalence in the mother–child relationship was achieved with the help of an alliance with the therapist. To a certain extent both the pediatrician and the husband had already been able to serve in this way. However, G.'s mother had not been able to perceive the pediatrician as sufficiently helpful because she had developed a maternal transference to him in which she experienced him as controlling—and this only intensified her ambivalence. Only as a result of her reflection on her own relationship with her mother and the structuring of our relationship and arrangements, which were derived from this reflection, could she relax and thereby improve the mother–child interaction.

In spite of my offer to be available for further contact later, G.'s mother did not contact me. I therefore don't know whether new interactional disorders developed during later developmental phases.

~

## ATTACHMENT DISORDERS IN SCHOOL-AGE CHILDREN

The attachment disorders of infancy and early childhood that I have described can also appear during the school years. The symptoms differ at different ages, however, not only because separation is a prerequisite for going to school, but also because the problems that surround achievement and the onset of puberty, with its aggressiveness and sexuality, must be dealt with for the first time.

### School Phobias

*Initial Presentation and Symptoms*

J.'s mother calls to set up psychotherapy for her son, who is almost 11. Her voice is urgent and upset. The boy is supposedly in his first year at a new school; however, except for the first 2 weeks of the school year, he has not attended classes in 3 months. I schedule an appointment right away. The mother cancels a few days later, however, because her son has been diagnosed with a bacterial stomach infection, which could explain the stomachaches he has had in connection with going to school. This illness has to be treated first. According to her, the father suffered through a similar illness with severe stomachaches.

Three months after this first phone call, the mother calls again and urgently requests another initial consultation. The situation has not changed at all, in spite of a variety of medical tests and even surgical intervention.

In the initial session, I encounter a very upset mother who is under a great deal of pressure—she races through her son's life story without so much as a comma or a period, but manages to do so in a very differentiated way and with great emotional involvement. The boy, by contrast, sits hunched up on a chair with his head bowed, looking downtrodden, with a mixture of apathy and depression. He takes no part in the conversation. I speak to him directly and encourage him to add to or correct his mother's information, but he rejects my advances, saying that his mother knows best.

The boy has not gone to school for almost half the year. With the support and guidance of his mother he has done all of his homework and diligently kept up with the material being covered in his classes. All attempts to bring him to school, however, have foundered on his stomachaches, and the nausea that includes gagging and vomiting. Over this period there have also been great changes in his behavior. Although he was once cheerful and outgoing, he has become increasingly withdrawn, sits around the house, and no longer participates in sports. He has become isolated and lonely. This distresses even him, so that he sometimes cries out his misery in his mother's arms. Everyone is at a loss.

## Patient History

The mother's report was highly reflective, and she talks fluently. J. is the second of two sons, his brother being 6 years older. He also attends a middle school, and there have been no problems with him. She describes her pregnancy and the boy's birth and early childhood development as completely unremarkable. According to the mother, he had been a lively, curious, and cheerful child. He had no trouble achieving good grades in primary school, and for this reason no one thought it necessary to discuss his transition to the middle school. However, a few days after entering the new school, he complained that he felt ill; first he reported nausea and stomachaches, and then he vomited. His mother could not bring herself to send him to school "in such a condition." A variety of physical tests were done in search of the cause of his illness, and finally a bacterial stomach infection was diagnosed and treated with high-dose antibiotics. J.'s complaints abated for several days, but then the symptoms resumed unchanged. At this point a surgeon was consulted. He diagnosed an umbilical hernia, and outpatient corrective surgery was performed. Characteristically, the pains decreased for several days after the operation, and the boy went to school for 2 hours on a trial basis. However, he became ill again and had to be picked up. After that the mother gave up her half-time job to care for her son's physical needs at home and to help him with his schoolwork. The father had been traveling on business a great deal, and the question arose whether J. might have been infected by the father with some tropical virus or other exotic illness. The next step under consideration is comprehensive testing at an institute for tropical diseases. The mother spends a great deal of time with this son; the 17-year-old has largely separated and is not home much.

The mother feels completely overwhelmed by the situation. Neither tests nor treatments have brought about any symptomatic change, and she has seen her son become depressed and withdrawn, which disturbs her greatly. In her excessive caregiving, she has absorbed all of her son's emotions and changes. Thus, she brought with her to our second meeting a notebook containing a detailed "document" in which she had recorded the course of his illness, tracked by date and intensity, and including even the slightest changes in symptoms.

When I ask her for more information, I learn that J. greatly fears a particular female teacher at school, whom he had experienced as strict, unfair, and very demanding during those first 2 weeks. He confirms this when I talk with him; I am also told that he has not integrated himself into the class at all. He does, however, have a good friend who is in the same class, but this contact has broken off almost completely because of his illness. It was very difficult for J. to get used to so many new students; all the new faces disturbed and frightened him. He also experienced the new teachers, whose behavior he could not predict, as more or less threatening.

During a projective test based on picture stories about the adventures of a little pig, the boy's associations focused on going out into the wide world and exploring. He expressed the fantasy that if he separated from the family, his mother might forget him if he wandered off too far.

### Consideration of Attachment Dynamics

From a classical psychodynamic perspective, it appears that J. has a symbiotically close relationship to his mother, who cares for him excessively. His transfer to the middle school in town, and the separation from his mother associated with it, leads to anxiety that expresses itself at a psychosomatic level as school phobia. His wishes for independence, as J. fantasizes them in a projective test, are split off, because he unconsciously fears that his mother might forget him if he were to go out into the world. His symptoms ensure that separation from the mother will not occur. However, because the parents do not understand the psychodynamics, they look for somatic causes of the stomachaches, involving a wide array of tests and treatments including even surgery. Clarification of the oedipal relationship with the father has not been very successful because he is often away, and he is therefore largely unavailable. In the transference to the female teacher whom J. experiences as so demanding and rejecting, the ambivalent relationship to the mother is replayed. J. wants to establish boundaries in his relationship with the teacher, but he fears his aggressive impulses, which in the transference are really meant for the mother.

From the perspective of attachment dynamics, however, it appears that J. has an ambivalent and controlling–caregiving attachment to his mother, who emanates powerful attachment needs vis-à-vis J. As a result, she relates to J. in a way that is inappropriate for his age, and she worries about every little vicissitude of his emotional and somatic development, acting as a sort of hypersensitive regulator. The mother is not very aware of J.'s needs for exploration and autonomy. It is additionally possible that the boy represents a secure base for the mother when the father is on his business trips, which last for several weeks. The school situation, and the possibilities for exploration and self-reliance that it represents, cannot be successfully negotiated given the existing insecure attachment relationship because, although J. wants greater autonomy, he fears that his mother will not allow it. All of the medical tests, and the entire home setup, including J.'s refusal to go to school and his mother's direct caregiving, demonstrate how much mother and son need each other in their entangled ambivalence. The mother had taken some steps to "individuate" within the family as the children got older; now, however, she has given up her part-time job to stay home and take care of her sick son. This, too, can only be understood as the mother's own ambivalence in the face of her unconscious fear of autonomy and exploration.

*Therapy and Course*

The parents still believed that a tropical virus was the most likely cause of their son's illness, and they were only willing to consider psychodynamics as a secondary possibility, so a final round of inpatient diagnostic tests was agreed to by all. Psychotherapy with J. and counseling with the parents were undertaken in the inpatient medical setting with the cooperation of the pediatrician, the goal being to enable the boy to go back to school.

The required tests, including blood tests, were completed in 2 days, and the findings were discussed at a meeting of the colleagues treating the somatic symptoms, the parents, and me. An organic cause of the symptoms was ruled out in view of the numerous preliminary tests. The parents pressed for gastrointestinal studies as a "final test," but since there was no evidence of gastrointestinal illness, we were able to dissuade them from this course. Instead we shared with them our psychodynamic perspective. We advised them that, in our assessment, the boy wanted greater autonomy, and that he viewed his new school situation with curiosity as an opportunity to explore and develop, but that at the same time he continued to feel closely attached to his mother. The mother reported that J. had always been her problem child and that it was true that she found it hard to "give him freedom." For this reason, the son always slept in the mother's bed while the father was traveling. Although I recognized these oedipal aspects, I did not place them in the foreground. In order to ease the son's ambivalent relationship with the mother, we considered whether the father might be able to arrange his professional schedule for a while so that he could take the boy to school in the morning.

At the time, J. could not imagine getting on the bus to go to school, either alone or with friends. Even though he vigorously opposed being taken to school by his father, and though he could hardly imagine not getting stomachaches, we carried out this plan on a trial basis. Because the father was considerably clearer and more structured than his wife in his relationship with their son, he foresaw no problem in picking him up at the hospital clinic in the morning and taking him to school. For the first several days J. insisted that his father accompany him to the classroom. (The teacher had been informed of this plan.) He complained to his father of stomachaches and nausea at first, although these were less evident in the clinic.

J. couldn't sleep on the third day, and he woke up with nausea and a stomachache. Because the treatment team and the parents were now increasingly convinced that the symptoms had a psychodynamic basis, the boy was given a hot water bottle but was required to go to school that morning. Accompanied by his father, he attended school as planned, even though he felt ill. Once there, his father "pushed" him through the door, and the teacher greeted him in a friendly manner. He was able to follow the lessons and did not have to cut the day short. He was also accepted by his classmates.

After 2 weeks there was another meeting with son and parents to discuss the progress that had been made as well as the difficulties encountered. We were able to plan J.'s discharge from the clinic so that the father's role in the therapy could be continued from home. Discharge was followed by a period of individual outpatient treatment for the son and intensive counseling for the mother. I offered to talk to her on difficult mornings after the boy had left the house. It was clear during these telephone calls that the mother could barely tolerate her son's complaints about stomachaches and nausea, so little could she disentangle herself from him emotionally. On the whole, however, J.'s school attendance stabilized. His relationship with his father and their activities together, which included crafts and motorcycling, were the main focus of his individual sessions. He no longer mentioned school phobia or stomachaches. Intensive individual counseling for the mother with occasional couples meetings continued on an outpatient basis. By then, the mother could think about starting to work again, and this led to a general relaxation of the situation. As a result of the sense of security gained during counseling, J.'s mother was able to engage with her own exploratory process. This included acceptance of her son and other family members as separate individuals, and embracing more autonomy and self-reliance for herself. J. was a talented boy and soon was sufficiently integrated into school that he could participate successfully in his class work. In spite of an absence of almost 6 months, he completed the year successfully because his mother had worked through the subject matter with him at home while he was ill.

### Concluding Remarks and Follow-Up

This intervention, founded in attachment theory and strengthened by the father's participation, both supported the son's wish for exploration and autonomy in the presence of a high level of ambivalence while at the same time loosening his pathologically entangled attachment to his mother.

The triadic mother–father–son relationship can also be interpreted from an oedipal perspective. J.'s oedipal conflicts had not been dealt with up to that time, and the father's task was to extricate the son from the ambivalent attachment relationship with the mother.

J. had a successful school year and was promoted, which made him very proud. He also took up sports again with his club. According to his mother, his behavior toward her was increasingly aggressive and adolescent. This became a subject of discussion in the individual sessions with J., which were taking place at increasingly greater intervals; he complained that his mother treated him "like a baby," which embarrassed him in front of his friends and teammates.

It was important to explain this change in J.'s behavior to his mother, both in terms of the onset of puberty and with regard to the aggressive components associated with ambivalent attachment. The mother was very relieved that J.'s behavior was "completely normal" and that she doesn't have to worry but can now "take care of myself more."

## Underachievement

*Initial Presentation and Symptoms*

I receive a telephone call from a couple whose 14-year-old son, M., is about to be suspended from school. The mother, who is quite upset, tells me that this event was preceded by several school transfers. Now M. must leave his present school, which means that he will not graduate with his class. For years M. simply has not participated in school; he sits with his head on the desktop for hours on end, doesn't get involved in class, and has become very withdrawn, unapproachable, and close-mouthed.

*Patient History*

M. was the couple's first child. He was followed by two sisters, 2 and 4 years younger. The sisters are very successful in school and go their own way. M., however, has always been a problem child, particularly for the mother. In spite of the aptitude he has demonstrated on all the school tests, he consistently holds himself back, remaining silent and aloof in school. He refuses to do his homework or participate in class. He has repeated this pattern in several schools. The mother is now despairing. She wonders whether she will be able to find a way out for her son.

During our initial consultation M. is taciturn and sullen. He claims not to understand why he is even there. Yes, he wants help—but then again he doesn't. In the countertransference I experience him as distant, withdrawn, and rejecting, but at the same time very troubled; as he says, himself, he constantly gets stuck "in the same pattern." While talking to the parents alone, I learn that the mother had been in treatment for her own anxiety symptoms several years before.

She recalls that all transitions (preschool, elementary school, junior high school) had been associated with considerable problems. M. had always preferred to withhold himself, so that from the very beginning she had to spend a good deal of time "setting him on the right path." The parents are distressed about his behavior because success is highly regarded by the entire family.

*Consideration of Attachment Dynamics*

All attempts to motivate M. to participate in school with behavioral therapy have failed. M. consistently gravitates to the same pattern, provoking suspension from school for noneffort, with subsequent school transfer. The mother has been intensively involved with him during the entire time. However, her efforts to motivate M. to adopt different behavior have been unsuccessful as well. Over the years a very intense relationship between mother and son has been built as a result. The beginnings of the age-appropriate desire for autonomy associated with puberty were not yet in evidence. Although the mother is in a better position to handle anxiety and separation now as a result of her own treatment, she concedes that her son may be less able to do so.

My understanding of attachment theory leads me to believe that M. has a close, ambivalent attachment to his mother. His nonparticipation in school enables him to maintain this intense attachment; at the same time, it lets him bring his fantasies about aggression and autonomy that are bound up with it into the interaction nonverbally. Autonomy may be made more difficult as well by M.'s disinclination to identify with his father, who is very dedicated to his profession. His lack of effort within a family that is highly performance-oriented guarantees high levels of attention from his mother.

I suspect that it will be necessary in therapy to promote the son's age-appropriate exploration and autonomy and the activities connected with them, while at the same time supporting the mother in her ability to recognize her son as an individual. For the time being, how helpful the father is in supporting this strategy is an open question.

*Therapy and Course*

M. was sullen when he arrived for individual therapy. Sessions consisted primarily of small-talk because he didn't "want to talk about anything else." He tended to be monosyllabic. In the countertransference, it was very difficult to tolerate his way of relating by means of silence. I did learn that M. occasionally fears that he might drop dead. He breathes much too quickly when he has such fantasies. He has had several acute anxiety attacks in the past. Once he even had to end a vacation and return home alone with his mother. These diffuse feelings of anxiety and psychosomatic fears, which are often associated with a "nervous heart" or anxiety neurosis, most recently occurred when M. was about to get on a cable lift. Working through this scene, with the accompanying images of leaving all his family members behind, plunging and crashing (the attachment of the car to the cable could break), and dying, led to intensive processing of his wish for and anxiety about autonomy. Over the entire course of his individual therapy, which took place at M.'s request sometimes weekly and sometimes every 2 weeks, his parents, and especially his mother, were drawn into the treatment. In my individual conversations with the parents, and occasionally alone with the mother, we focused on her anxieties surrounding her son's individuation and the significance of the father as a figure of identification for him.

M. became increasingly able to enter into relations with his circle of friends. He now more frequently went to parties and discos at night. At first, the mother was very anxious about this and had trouble sleeping until her son "finally" got home. We discussed this scenario for a fairly long time because in it the close entwinement between mother and son was clearly evident. Over time M. came to understand the entangled nature of attachment with his mother and that, although he wanted to become more autonomous, this aroused considerable anxiety, including the fear of death.

At the same time, M. was continuing his studies at an evening school, which he attended regularly and quite successfully. The lack of effort described earlier no longer occurred. He was also demonstrating more self-reliant behavior. The high point of the individuation process occurred when the parents planned a summer vacation out of the country for several weeks, and M. simply refused to go along with them. He was far more interested in structuring his own vacations with his friends and planning outings, camping, and other activities. I had to support the mother emotionally so that she could go on her vacation in spite of her anxiety at not knowing exactly what her son might be up to during her absence. M. did have an accident during his vacation and had to be admitted for inpatient treatment; however, he had no permanent injuries. The fact that he coped with everything without his mother, and that his mother "survived it," placed a heavy burden on the mother–son relationship. This experience, after all, embodied both the mother's and son's fears that increasing exploration and independence were linked to fatal dangers and risks. The experience of overcoming these risks represented clear progress in therapy.

It was also important for M. to be mobile—that is, to "have wheels"—so that he could get around in a manner appropriate to his age without having to depend on "Mom's Taxi." Because of their common interest in motorcycles, M. found a new topic of conversation with his father, which intensified his identification with him.

*Concluding Remarks and Follow-Up*

M. was able to make a good start on the process of individuation and autonomy. This might not have been possible but for the mother's attachment-oriented therapy that took place in tandem with his. Because M.'s mother was able to experience therapy as a secure base, she was eventually able to endure her son's steps toward autonomy. Simultaneously M. stopped experiencing fantasied separation as potentially life-threatening, and he was able to engage in age-appropriate interaction within his group of teenaged friends.

# Aggressiveness

The most significant characteristic of this attachment disorder is that aggressive behavior can serve to establish and maintain attachment. If this attachment dynamic is not understood, aggressive behavior (in school, for example) will be met with punishment. If neither the need for attachment nor the way it is expressed is understood, the result may be an attenuation of the attachment between teacher and child, thus leading to intensification of the disturbing behavior.

### Initial Presentation and Symptoms

Eight-year-old T.'s parents contact me at his teacher's urging. T. creates disturbances in class almost constantly—he is provocative, can't keep still, hits other children, and is "almost impossible to keep in class." His parents are completely baffled, because at home their son is well integrated into the family and into his circle of friends in the neighborhood and doesn't demonstrate the aggressive and provocative behaviors the teacher describes.

### Patient History

The parents don't understand why T., who has up to now caused them no problems, should begin to act so aggressively after changing teachers in third grade. The parents blame the teacher for T.'s behavior; they feel that she does not structure her class well enough and is unable to control the students. They feel all the more justified in this opinion because T.'s behavior is not at all conspicuous at home. This discrepancy has caused considerable tension between the parents and the teacher, who feels that the parents don't understand her. The parents are of the opinion that the teacher needs pedagogical counseling.

T. was the only child, and because the mother worked only in the morning, she could help him with his homework or other activities if he wanted. Supposedly, however, T. mainly played in the street with his friends and was "completely happy."

### Consideration of Attachment Dynamics

Given his behavior at home and the fact that no difficulties had appeared during the past school years, it may be assumed that T. has had a secure attachment to his parents. Now T. is attempting to establish a relationship with the new teacher; he is frustrated in these attempts, however, because she is new to the class and is completely overloaded by having to build relationships with all the many unfamiliar children. It might have been helpful if T. had already developed a secure attachment to his class so that group attachment could have replaced or bridged the attachment that had not yet developed to his new teacher. However, it is clear that his attachment to the group is not yet strong enough, and that T. is dependent on his new teacher as an individual attachment figure in school. By expressing his anger and disappointment at not having his needs for support met by engaging in aggressive behavior, he ensures prompt attention so that his wish for attachment is reinforced at this level of behavior. Over time, however, his behavior leads to withdrawal on the teacher's part, and a vicious cycle develops.

A classical dynamic view might lead one to wonder if T. has a negative transference to the new teacher. But the patient's history gives us few indications of what aspects of the teacher's behavior might have triggered such a negative transference.

*Therapy and Course*

At the parents' request and with the teacher's consent, we scheduled a meeting with both parties. I reported that T. is very well adapted and well-behaved during individual play sessions with me. This did not surprise the teacher because, after all, T. has individual contact with me and is not part of a group. I concurred with her view and supported her idea that his behavior in the group is certainly more difficult because, given the class size, he has to compete with many other children for her attention. The teacher reports that she is constantly busy dealing with the commotion he creates, his running around and his provocative behavior, and that often she spends half the class time trying to get T. under control. Twice she has had to make him stay after school, after which he became amazingly cooperative. In fact, he looked forward to staying after, something she couldn't understand. Normally children talk during this time or try to evade it. She fears that T. may continue to disturb the classroom in order to have the "pleasure" of staying after school.

On closer questioning, it turned out that T.'s teacher had taken over a very large class with many active, and even hyperactive, children, and that she felt herself stretched beyond her capacities in trying to structure the class and establish attachment relationships with so many children. She felt particularly overloaded, compromised, and rejected as a result of the aggressive and provocative behavior, which she felt unable to deal with.

Over the course of several further conversations, we pursued questions of attachment dynamics. Like all children in class, T. sought contact with and attachment to his new teacher. Obviously, his disturbing and aggressive style of behavior was well-suited to engage the teacher in interacting with and relating to him alone. I considered T.'s positive reaction to staying after school as a sign of his unconscious wish to establish a very personal attachment relationship with the teacher. This perspective was new to the parents as well, and they were relieved that their son had not become a bad and aggressive child who was headed for expulsion. We thought of the idea of having the teacher "stay after school" with T. twice a week for half an hour, but that these sessions should be scheduled independent of whether he had provoked her or not. By the time of our next meeting 3 weeks later, she had completely resolved her problem with T.'s aggressive behavior. He was friendly and engaged with the teacher during their "special time," and he showed her his best side. He was now motivated and cooperative in class, supporting the teacher and acting like a model of class participation. However, now the problem was how to create a transition for T. from this individualized attention back into the group, since the teacher was not prepared to give him such attention long-term. We held another meeting together with T., and we talked about his wish for attachment to the teacher. T. was very relieved that he was no longer seen as a bad boy who only caused trouble and had to be sent to stand in the corner. Because his attachment to the teacher had become more secure in the meantime, he did not appear to take it too hard that the individualized "after-school sessions" would be reduced and eventually ended. He now felt that his teacher appreciated him for his positive contributions and that his relationship with her had improved in spite of the competition from the other students.

*Concluding Remarks and Follow-Up*

This case of an aggressively troublesome student demonstrates that "time outs" and sending the child to stand in the corner, both of which increase distance and threaten termination of relationship, do not lead to a solution of the problem but actually intensify the undesirable behavior in cases where a wish for attachment lies behind the aggressive behavior. If treatment is to succeed, everyone must understand the attachment-related issues involved and must be drawn into a therapeutic alliance based on this understanding. Without attachment-oriented intervention, the relationship between the teacher and T. would probably have continued to worsen. Although individualized play therapy would have satisfied T.'s attachment needs, there had never been a deficiency in this area that would have led to such a problem at home in his attachment to the parents. I suspect that if he had been treated in an individual play therapy that satisfied his needs for attachment and emotional support, he would have adapted very cooperatively, but that his behavior toward the teacher would have stayed the same.

There were no problems over the rest of the school year. T. became a diligent and interested student who was much appreciated by his teacher.

~

## ATTACHMENT DISORDERS IN ADOLESCENCE

Attachment and self-reliance have particular significance in adolescence. Age-appropriate autonomy vis-à-vis parents is more easily negotiated when secure attachment has been achieved. When it has not, there are often disturbances in the individuation process.

### Addictive Symptoms

The following example examines in light of attachment theory the addictions so often seen in adolescents. It describes how substance dependency—in this case, on many types of drugs—can coexist with addictive relationships. These varying forms of addiction are not necessarily present in combination. The progression from romantic obsession with certain stars or music groups to disturbances involving addictive or very symbiotic relationships is a fluid one.

### Initial Presentation and Symptoms

Seventeen-year-old S. came to me, accompanied by a staff member from the child welfare office, after several police raids had found her drunk or in possession of small amounts of drugs. She repeatedly told the welfare workers that her troubles were the fault of her 30-year-old "friend," who often walked out on her and took up with other women. If he loved her the way she wanted, she would not have to drink alcohol or take drugs; she would be in seventh heaven without them.

S., at the initial consultation, is a well-dressed young woman wearing a good deal of makeup. She attempts to establish contact with me with small talk—"So, how's it going, and what can I do for you?"— thereby reversing our roles. She is clearly making an effort to present herself as autonomous and independent; she does not want to reveal any chinks in her armor or ask for advice or help. Her skillful chit-chat maneuvers me into the role of the one seeking help.

### Patient History

S. tells her family history as if it were a novel: exciting, dynamic, and creative, with many colorful examples.

She is the only child of rich parents. She has no idea where in the world they are currently traveling; she hasn't had regular contact with them for 2 years. She lives in a group home at the moment. She thinks that she may have been artificially conceived and that her father may not be her natural father. But that is unimportant. You can't depend on men anyway, so why should she give any thought to who her natural father is? Her mother spends all her time thinking about her own career, and as a child S. had been just another beautiful "ornament" to set out next to all the other museum pieces that her parents had collected. She had lacked for nothing—she had had an overabundance of toys and presents, and she had no idea how many nannies had taken care of her, or when they came or left. When one left, another was always available. She saw her mother occasionally for brief periods when they would make special excursions to the zoo or the movies, and so on. She always looked forward to these highlights, but somehow she always ended up disappointed because even when her mother spent an entire afternoon with her she was "never really there." When I asked S. what she meant by that, she answered defensively, "You know, being there, heart and soul."

S. first began to experience difficulties in adolescence, when she was constantly falling in love with different boys and could think of nothing else. According to her, school and learning were simply "passé." She was always bitterly disappointed in her relationships with boys and men because they were so undependable, and so she "sailed" from one to the next. I stay with this image and ask whether she has always looked for a harbor. S. becomes pensive and says, "Yes, you could look at it that way. Like a ship on the high seas, constantly discovering new exotic islands, losing oneself completely in fantasies. How wonderful it would be on these islands . . . except there is no harbor, no harbor where the boat could be anchored safe from the waves, or where one could make a homey and familiar place ashore."

Our dialogue branches out into philosophical matters, which the patient ornaments with quotations and examples from The Little Prince. She also mentions that her mother has married for the third time, and that S. is not exactly sure where she is. She has had no contact with her father for 2 years. She went to a number of private schools because of her academic problems, but she failed at each because, according to S., she always "fell fatally in love." At some point, out of frustration, she began to drink at parties; when she was drinking, her pain at being left by yet another boy was tolerable. She had her first sexual encounter at the age of 12, and sexually too she slid from one relationship to another. Again, I stay with her image and ask whether, when "sliding," she had ever wanted support. She became pensive again and said after a while, "Yes, support, being held, not being alone anymore, having someone who is always there for me. But those are silly fantasies that can never come true."

I sense clearly that she is becoming sad and thoughtful and withdrawing into herself. Eventually she reports that it was in such phases of depression that she first began to try drugs: never regularly but always when things got particularly bad and she could no longer endure her pain, grief, and yearning. I am surprised at how apparently openly, reflectively, and insightfully she is able to talk about herself.

### Consideration of Attachment Dynamics

S. traces her present problems to her unclear parentage. It is an open question whether or not she was really wanted and planned, or only served as a narcissistic display for her parents, but in any case she was never drawn into a real emotional attachment or relationship with them. A series of nannies had taken care of her, and at some point she had stopped hoping that any one of them might stay longer. Her contact with her mother, and their excursions, meant a great deal to her, but in the end she came to feel that this was a formal kind of contact with very little emotional significance. She looks for a "safe harbor" where she can drop anchor. It would hardly be possible to express a desire for attachment more clearly.

S. began in adolescence to try to realize this desire in a variety of relationships, including sexual ones, but these failed, in part because the boys of that age could not respond to the intensity of S.'s desire for attachment. This deeply disappointed her. Early attachment disappointments and the entire sweep of her grief about the attachment to her parents that she had not let herself feel came to the surface. Eventually, the pain became so great that she tried to suppress it with alcohol and drugs, or at least to make it tolerable. But the development of addiction did not blunt her attachment needs.

A dynamic is thus created in which the drug itself becomes a pseudo-secure attachment object that is supposed to take the place of genuine attachment. The drug is always there, always available; it comforts painful feelings and leaves behind it a sense of being supported and relaxed. It can be used as needed, and it can satisfy desires and needs for support, security, and dependability, which S. can regulate herself; needs for attachment and autonomy can be satisfied and handled flexibly, using the drug as a "surrogate." As long as it is available, the drug is more dependable than any human. It can run out, but conflicts around relationship dynamics or attachment difficulties are never held responsible, only the lack of money. Eventually, with her increasing drug dependency, the desire for attachment and friendship disappeared. The drug superficially satisfied all desires and needs.

These considerations point toward an avoidant attachment pattern. S.'s capacity to talk about herself introspectively is not consistent with this assessment because, over the course of therapy, it became clear that her facility in talking about herself, her needs, and her relational wants is superficial and not accompanied by any real conviction or feeling.

From a classical psychoanalytic perspective, one might see in this patient an oedipal conflict with her largely absent father, or perhaps unresolved oedipal issues in general. Her rejection by, and then of, her natural father and the search for relationships with older men that is a consequence, as well as the rapid and spontaneous transference relationship that occurred during our first two conversations, all speak for this. This dynamic is surely present, but in my diagnostic consideration and in my approach to therapy it is not central. Rather, I consider problems of attachment dynamics to be primary.

*Therapy and Course*

In contrast with the usual behavior of adolescents (including adolescents with quite advanced addictions who are hesitant about coming to therapy or even refuse to do so at all), S. said that she wanted to continue therapy after our first dialogues. She stated, however, that several sessions per week was out of the question for her.

A stormy transference relationship developed. From some perspectives, this might have been be interpreted as either an erotic or an oedipal transference, but from my perspective it was her primary unsatisfied wishes for attachment that were central to the transference.

S. was constantly frustrated and disappointed at the structuring of the setting and the limited number of sessions. These disappointments made it difficult for her not to "chuck" her treatment and search for a better or different therapist, or even quit completely. Precisely because her wishes were so excessive, and her attachment disorder so reminiscent of a pattern of social promiscuity, I did not give in to her desire to increase the frequency of therapy but, rather, kept it to 2 hours per week, sitting. In my experience, it is an error to try to satisfy too quickly the attachment hunger of such patients. No sufficiently secure base exists yet to allow them to tolerate disappointments and frustrations, and all too often the relationship is terminated quickly, even though provision for their needs has been made. Such patients then look for a new primary attachment object in the hope that the new one will be more reliable and will satisfy their unstillable attachment needs.

In this case, a therapeutic process developed in which I had to tolerate with great sensitivity the young woman's frustrations and disappointments, her rage, and her relentless wishes and demands. For a long time I felt in the countertransference as though I were perceived as a thing—interchangeable, used today and perhaps chucked aside tomorrow. S.'s affective reactions were very powerful. For considerable periods she oscillated between her intense desire for relationship and her termination fantasies. Only during the midphase of treatment, after 60 sessions, did I begin to experience a more stable relationship, in which I started to feel that I was being perceived as an interlocutor. There now began a clear phase of grief processing connected with the resolution of the vain hopes she had held out for her relationships with her mother, her father, and all of the nursemaids. She was now able to react with sadness, and greater relatedness, to the fact that her wish for more therapy and greater closeness would not be satisfied if she immediately reacted with threats or with fantasies about terminating therapy.

During this period, S. began to attend school again. However, a crisis developed when she reached the age where she could no longer live in the group home and would have to move out. With the help of the child welfare office she found a solution. Although she would continue to live alone, she would be looked after on an individual basis by a youth worker, who would provide home visits and support in negotiating day-to-day social demands. It was important to S. for the youth worker and me to maintain contact with each other and understand what the other was doing. In her fantasy, we became her substitute parents, and her most important attachment figures.

Issues of autonomy, exploration, and attachment came to play a role in her relationship with the youth worker, and also with me as her therapist. S. wanted the youth worker to visit less often, and increasingly wanted to decide and negotiate matters alone. Occasionally she missed therapy, and then, with embarrassment, telephoned me to apologize. During that phase of treatment, I saw this less as resistance than as the beginnings of autonomy.

*Concluding Remarks and Follow-Up*

S. made great efforts to continue treatment. In her fantasy, at least, it was never supposed to end; it should not terminate or be interrupted, which she considered "unnatural." She continued in school, and she graduated. She became increasingly more skilled at making her own decisions and planning her life. Even though she occasionally drank at parties or smoked a joint, she was no longer in acute danger of redeveloping a drug addiction or dependency. It is still an open question how much her behavior is a residual symptom, an unresolved problem relating to attachment and relationship, and how much it is an age-appropriate adolescent desire for pleasure and exploration.

S. began to develop longer-term partnerships and relationships. She was able to deal in a more constructive way with periods of grief without increasing her reliance on drugs. I received sporadic letters, postcards, or telephone calls from her—"signs of life." I answered them, and made myself available as a secure base in accord with the shifts in her desire for contact or distance. The danger of fusion, once so desired by her, no longer existed; that is, it had been possible to work through and resolve the transference without the permanent termination that would be required by other psychodynamic approaches.

## Antisocial Behavior and Delinquency

Antisocial behavior includes such manifestations as lying, stealing, running away, minor transgressions of rules and norms, truancy, and delinquency (including petty theft and even muggings), and is becoming increasingly widespread among adolescents.

*Initial Presentation and Symptoms*

Thirteen-year-old P. is sent by the court for psychiatric treatment after he has been arrested several times. He was known to attend school only sporadically, and he had come to the attention of the court because of frequent shoplifting, forged signatures, and attempted check fraud. He also took frequent "joyrides" in his father's high-horsepower car, and had once caused a high-speed accident that resulted in damages.

P. is a stocky, obstinate, and depressed-looking boy who comes to treatment unwillingly and resists admission to the clinic, even though he allowed himself to be taken to the unit "like a sacrificial lamb." He has already been schooled by his brushes with the law and the resulting interrogations, and all I can get out of him at our initial conversation is that he is innocent and misunderstood by everybody. If only the automobile accident hadn't happened, he wouldn't be here. His parents will pay the damages, so why should he be admitted for inpatient treatment? Automobile accidents like that happen every day, but not everybody who causes an accident is sent to see a psychiatrist.

P. is very glib, argumentative, and clever for his age, and he tries to defend himself by these means. Neither his life story nor any of the "charges" brought against him have anything to do with him. In the countertransference, I oscillate between annoyance, the desire to confront, and even to provoke, P. with his misdeeds, and a feeling of helplessness coupled with an impulse to turn him away. What am I supposed to do with this maladjusted adolescent who is just not interested in therapy? Any efforts on my part are bound to be wasted.

*Patient History*

P. is an only child. At the time of his inpatient admission, his father was not available, as he was serving time in prison on a variety of fraud charges. It was hard to persuade his mother, who works shifts, to come in for an initial consultation because, although she felt relieved that P. had been admitted as an inpatient, she also wanted to "fight for his release." As far as she can recall, she tells me, his early childhood development was unremarkable, but in fact she doesn't remember the details of her pregnancy, the birth, or his early development. She clearly resists remembering that time, letting me know that it is all in the past and, anyway, it isn't why she's here.

Apparently, P.'s difficulties began at puberty, when the boy was teased in school for being overweight. He stopped wanting to go to school, and often stayed home while his mother went to work. Over the past year he had spent days on end locked in the house with the blinds down. All attempts to lure him out of his "cave" went nowhere. During this period he had frequently sat in his father's car at night, and then one night he had driven off in it—his mother couldn't say how often he went on such expeditions. Then he got involved in the accident. Although the damages were serious, the family would pay.

P. was not "crazy," his mother told me, which was why she would fight for his release from the psychiatric unit. She made light of his previous thefts and swindles, including the check fraud. She spoke with great difficulty about the problems related to the father's imprisonment. P. had watched his father hide from the police until the day he was taken by surprise and arrested while trying to visit the family. P. had suffered greatly as a result of this, as his relationship with his father was very important to him. All contact with the father had been prohibited by the court, because the court "absurdly" believed that P. had been involved in the swindles and that his father had told him where considerable sums of money had been stashed.

## Consideration of Attachment Dynamics

I suspect that P.'s attachments are insecure and that neither his mother nor his father represent a secure base for him. His father's arrest weighs more heavily on him than the separation from his mother caused by the inpatient admission. This could indicate that P. is more ambivalently attached to his father than to his mother. Although he claims that he cannot survive without his mother, and that she wants to "fight" for him, at the emotional level it is hard to discern real attachment. I get the impression instead that the mother is fighting over P. so that she can keep him at home to satisfy her own attachment needs. It remains unclear whether the father is exploiting his relationship with P. for his fraudulent activities.

It is possible that P.'s reaction to his father's arrest was an intensified grief reaction: that he locked himself in his room, depressed, to mourn the loss of his father there. If so, he may have stopped being able to go

to school because his ego functioning was overtaxed by his intense reaction to the separation. Symbolically, the father's automobile helped the
boy to fantasize emotional closeness with his father; P. may feel emotionally connected to his father while driving his car. One thing is certain: P.'s desire and need for attachment was never satisfied in any way.
Over and over, even before the clinic admission, he had received more
attention through his interactions with the police and the child welfare
office than from his parents. An entire network of secondary caregivers
figures was concerned about him. Although his parents expressed care
indirectly to the extent of battling over relationship, they never demonstrated it in concrete, caring ways.

P.'s delinquent and antisocial behavior may be understood as an attempt to have his needs for care (which remain unsatisfied by his parents) addressed by social institutions, as represented by the child welfare office workers and judges. Seen in a larger context, society,
challenged by P.'s behavior, is asked to be a secure base with clearly
structured rules that can protect P. from his own impulses and tie him
into the social framework.

## Therapy and Course

The treatment setting consisted of individual therapy twice a week and
group therapy three times weekly. This schedule was established on the
grounds that P. would be more able to risk age-appropriate relationships
with a peer group in group therapy if he first developed some emotional
security in individual therapy. P. was seen as something of a loner who
avoided contact with others on the unit and who made arrangements
about many things for himself alone. Although he did show up more or
less punctually and willingly for his individual sessions during the initial phase, he was obstinate and sullen during the sessions, gave inso-
lent responses, and clearly resisted treatment. In the group, in contrast,
he kept very quiet. There, he was withdrawn and avoided relationships,
even with his designated support figures on the unit, while acting
extraordinarily well-behaved and well-adjusted at the same time. It
would have been easy to forget that he was there.

On the unit, P. was showing us the other side—the well-behaved
and well-adjusted side—of his personality. He plodded along, appar-

ently without emotional desire or need for attachment and relationship. His behavior was such that there was no reason to continue treating him on an inpatient basis—superficially, at least. I argued, however, that from the perspective of attachment dynamics an enormous emotional neediness (indicated by hanging out in his father's car, stealing it, engaging in the same kind of criminal behavior) might be hidden behind his aloof behavior in the group.

This set the stage for our individual sessions, where P. with increasingly regularity used therapy to discuss everyday issues, such as time off and privileges. Finally, we found a topic that filled many hours. P. was very knowledgeable about automobiles and racing, and he could talk for hours on all manner of details in this area. An outsider might view this as resistance: by talking about automobiles he avoided his own feelings. From the point of view of attachment dynamics, however, I understood that he had gained enough emotional security in his individual therapy to talk about the difficult situation he faced in his relationship with his father— through the topic "automobile." At first, I said nothing to him about this. Only after many hours, and again by means of a discussion of the technical details, were we able to talk about his father's car, which P. had turned into scrap. His relationship with his father was not yet a subject of explicit discussion; P. simply ignored any attempt to talk about his father directly. He attended group therapy at the same time, where, although he didn't talk about emotional matters, he was now recognized and valued by the other adolescents for his technical knowledge.

Staff members noted that after group sessions P. and the others went to the canteen, where he would stock up on sweets, which he devoured indiscriminately. I understood this to be another expression of his attachment desires and needs, although in the classical literature it would have been interpreted as regression to the oral phase. In my view, P. was attempting to regulate the emotional needs and depressive feelings (stemming originally from his early development, and activated in therapy) with sweets and oral gratification. Only after many more hours did P. become able to talk about his desire to visit his father in prison. This confirmed my assumption that the father was P.'s primary attachment figure.

I handled this wish very concretely, discussing with the court and the legal authorities how such a visit might be made possible. P. was almost transformed after his first visit to his father. He was considerably less depressed and more lively, and he participated actively in the life of the unit. A short while later, with tears in his eyes, he was able to talk about his father in group therapy for the first time. The fear that he had fantasized about in individual therapy—that the group would laugh at and ostracize him—proved unfounded. The group reacted with great sensitivity and sympathy, and was impressed by how he handled his situation. This strengthened his attachment to his peer group, and so the group, as well as his individual therapy, became an important secure base from which and with which to explore his inner and outer world. At first P. had observed the unit rules with docility; later he resisted the rules, either ignoring or breaking them. Now he was considerably more able to observe the unit framework and negotiate free time and special privileges with reference figures. All in all, he had become much more capable of establishing relationships.

There followed a phase of intense effort to draw the mother into the treatment with regular family sessions. So far, she had either come to appointments late or had canceled them on short notice. P. finally realized that the wish for involvement that his mother repeatedly expressed did not correspond to reality; she consistently used other important matters and appointments so as not to have to visit him. It took a great deal of effort and many confrontations to move the mother in the direction of a somewhat more reliable relationship, and the effort was not particularly successful. In his individual therapy, P. engaged in grief work, which, with his now-secure attachment base, he could now allow himself to do. He recognized that the desire for emotional support that he directed toward his mother was much more likely to be fulfilled by his father—but that his father was now unavailable, except during very limited visiting hours. For a long time P. vacillated between whether to return to his mother or look into the possibility of a group home. He was eventually discharged and went home, at his and his mother's request.

### Concluding Remarks and Follow-Up

As subsequent outpatient treatment showed, P. was now able to set clearer boundaries with his mother and keep himself from being drawn to such an extent into her emotional neediness. The experience he gained in the therapy group was of such significance that, after discharge, he was relatively quickly able to connect with a group of peers, who offered him a more secure base for his future development than his mother could. During his inpatient admission, which lasted almost a year, P. had also stabilized his academic work, and he was subsequently able to attend school regularly and graduate.

Neither during his subsequent outpatient treatment nor over the follow-up period that came after that did P. exhibit antisocial behavior. He was eventually able to begin an apprenticeship. His relationship with his mother continued to be distant, but he was no longer as dependent on her for reliable satisfaction of his attachment needs. Instead, he was sufficiently able to satisfy his needs for attachment through group, allowing him to explore the world as an adolescent with other adolescents. He maintained his important relationship with his father with regular prison visits.

## Neurodermatitis

Severe psychosomatic illnesses among adolescents, such as neurodermatitis, anorexia nervosa, bulimia, Crohn's disease, and ulcerative colitis place a great strain on family members. Severe physical symptoms often demand somatic treatment in parallel with psychotherapy, and may include monitoring of blood values, weight fluctuations, and so on. An adolescent in circumstances such as these is tied into a treatment regime that may satisfy his attachment needs, but not his wish for autonomy. From an attachment theory perspective, it is the therapist's task to help these adolescents find a helpful balance between attachment and autonomy.

*Initial Presentation and Symptoms*

Mr. O. calls and asks in a subdued and timid voice whether he can do therapy with me. He doesn't exactly know what "therapy" is; his family doctor referred him to me. He says that he has many problems, but that he can't talk about them on the phone.

A very tall, slim, 19-year-old man, his head pulled between his shoulders as he enters the door, comes to the initial consultation. Timidly he takes only my fingertips as we shake hands. I notice that he has a bandage on his left hand. He looks at me through his steel-rimmed glasses with a mixture of distrust and expectation. He waits for a long time until I finally take the initiative and begin to ask him questions.

He tells me that he's coming now because he has major problems with his girlfriend. She's actually very nice; she takes care of him, and he gets along with her quite well; the day-to-day relationship is not a problem. They have been living together for 6 months. Although he had yearned for this, he finds that he often can't endure being with her. He becomes aggressive and has to leave the apartment because he fears an "explosion." Violent thoughts like this come to him particularly when they are "very close," or being intimate with each other. He is very unhappy about this and doesn't know what to do. His girlfriend interprets his behavior as rejection, which makes him very sad. He has had skin problems for many years, and they have recently "blossomed." Because his skin is "open and bloody" in many areas, he is currently unable to work.

*Patient History*

Mr. O. was the eighth and last child in a very large family. He himself believes that his mother "had actually had enough after six." He remembers the names, ages, and birthdays of his siblings only with a great deal of effort, and he is not at all sure whether what he says is correct. He states that everything in his life has been very chaotic, and that his mother had been completely overburdened by her many children. He remembers his family as a place where everyone had to fight for his own survival.

He had skin problems even when he was an infant. His earliest recollections revolve around the daily fights he had with his mother when he was a preschooler because he did not want to let her put ointment on him. But his yelling and screaming were useless: "With my mother, you didn't have a chance."

When his skin problems got particularly bad during puberty, he had several long inpatient admissions for cortisone treatments. He remembers his time in the hospital as having been very pleasant. He particularly recalled an older nurse whose care for him had been especially loving. He always preferred to have her rub ointment on his skin.

He had a hard time graduating from school because he missed so much class time due to his illness. At present he is in an apprenticeship, but he is not sure whether he will be able to complete it because of his skin problems. He tells me also that he had a "special relationship" with his 4-year-older sister. "That," he says, "is a story all its own."

Over the course of the dialogue, Mr. O. speaks ever more softly and incoherently, in fragmentary phrases, and I can feel his sadness and pensiveness increase. In spite of his physical size, he actually shrivels in the chair. In the countertransference, I have an image of a little injured boy who needs many kinds of care.

*Consideration of Attachment Dynamics*

As the eighth and probably unwanted child, Mr. O.'s relationship with his mother is likely to have been very ambivalent right from the beginning. If one assumes that neurodermatitis has many causes, then one can at least speculate that an insecure attachment to the mother might be one aggravating co-factor. We may suspect that the mother experienced feelings of aggression and powerlessness toward the son who, as an infant, had resisted with such vehemence her daily attempts to put ointment on his skin. Also, presumably, the child would have felt this care to his raw skin as very painful, and himself at the mercy of his mother's actions and emotions. Although caregiving may be an activity that fosters attachment to the mother, this type of care in the face of vehement protest is also a very aggressive interaction. Mr. O.'s mother represented the place where he could hope to receive care, relief, and protection for his painful skin. However, he also must have hated her for the pain she occasioned in her insensitive disregard of his wild protest.[5] Such disregard for the child's needs in a situation that provokes fear leads to the experience of powerless rage and helplessness. This picture is typical of the disorganized attachment pattern.

I speculate that Mr. O.'s relationship to his mother was molded by a mixture of disorganized attachment with an underlying mixture of ambivalent and avoidant patterns. However, his ability to relate was evident in the fact that he felt emotional relief during his periods of inpatient treatment, and was apparently able to establish a positive relationship with an older nurse, allowing her to care for him without the aggressiveness that characterized his relationship with his mother. Perhaps his older sister may have served as his secure attachment figure. At the beginning of therapy, however, I was not at all clear what he meant by the "special relationship" with his sister.

It was remarkable that Mr. O.'s father did not appear at all in his entire narrative; when I inquired, the patient shrugged his shoulders and stated that his father "was always working." It remains unclear to me whether the father was present at all in the family. I suspect that the patient was so concerned with himself and his mother that in other respects he "disappeared" into the sibling group and was not sufficiently seen as an individual by the father.

Because of the difficult, entangled, and aggressively loaded nature of Mr. O.'s attachment relationship with his mother, I expect that he will demand a great deal of closeness and security as well as caregiving and support from me in therapy. However, it will also be important to recognize his need for distance, given his background of avoidant attachment.

*Therapy and Course*

During the first phase of therapy Mr. O. expressed a great deal of concern about his relationship with his girlfriend. He feared that he might lose her; but in spite of his intense desire and need for closeness, he could only tolerate closeness for short periods of time.

Mr. O. came to therapy three times a week, a frequency that he chose himself. He looked forward to the sessions, always arrived early, and came through the door beaming. It soon became clear, however, that a 50-minute session would be too long for him at first. He tested out sitting and lying down, and chose the lying position because he could relax better that way and didn't always have to look at me. In the classical psychoanalytic setting the therapist sits behind the patient, but at Mr. O.'s request I sat next to him because he felt that this did not threaten him or make him frightened. He could relax on the couch and look at me from time to time as needed. I was supposed to be with him in his feelings, but not (his great fear) "ambush him from behind": he recalled difficult encounters with his mother, who would "ambush" and catch him in the evening and then forcibly undress and bathe him before applying the ointment to his body, a procedure that seemed to him to last an eternity.

In the beginning there were times when he would have to get up after 20 minutes because he felt that he could no longer tolerate the tension inside him. Sometimes he would sit on the couch for a while, and sometimes we were able to continue working like that. However, he sometimes had to leave before the end of the session. Mr. O. said he felt guilty because he was using "my expensive time" three times a week, but then leaving before the end of the session, thereby disappointing me. In the context of his difficult attachment to his mother, we were able to talk about just how important it might be for him to decide for himself how much closeness or distance he needed. Over time, he was able to tolerate the physical tension he felt lying on the couch for longer periods.

During the phases of therapy when Mr. O. was looking at his enormous rage toward his mother, murderous fantasies began to appear of which he felt very ashamed. During this time, he experienced me as a persecutor who had forced him into "this stupid therapy" and who could determine everything, including date, time of session, beginning and end of session, and vacations. Any attempt to address his aggression and disparagement of me in the transference was met with even more vehement verbal attacks.

Only much later did I learn that during this time, filled with aggressive tension, he occasionally rode his motorcycle on dangerous winding roads. At times he would pass other vehicles at blind spots on the road, fantasizing that only a "huge explosion" could free him. These quasi-suicidal actions may be understood as an expression of his enormous early experiences of aggression. At this same time, his skin symptoms became so acute that he considered checking into the clinic again. He expressed fear that I would not be able to stand him with his "burst and bloody skin" and that sooner or later I would send him away, just the way his girlfriend had threatened to leave him.

It took a fair amount of time before he was able to discuss closeness and distance with his girlfriend: although it was good that she was there, he could not tolerate the sort of intense closeness that she wanted with him. Their relationship relaxed somewhat when he dared to discuss this topic with her and asked to be permitted to set the terms of closeness. It was not easy to get his girlfriend to understand that his withdrawal or distancing did not mean that he rejected her; quite the contrary. He felt well taken care of by her, but he sometimes felt fear of dependency.

Later in the treatment Mr. O.'s relationship to his older sister became very important. I understood that she had represented his most stable attachment figure. However, this attachment relationship was not without ambivalence. He told me that when he was going through puberty his sister would climb into his bed at night. He looked forward to these nightly visits and awaited his sister longingly, because he found closeness and physical contact with her under the covers to be very pleasant. However, at the same time he felt sexually pressured by her: "If I wanted to be close to her, I had to pay a price."

Now we could understand how this "special relationship" had been activated in the transference to his girlfriend and why he "exploded" at his girlfriend specifically in intimate situations.

Given his early rage, it required a high degree of sensitivity to follow and evaluate his desire for closeness and presence as well as for distance and attachment avoidance. Often I did not know what to do; I felt that his demands for closeness and security were balancing on a tightrope with his aggression and his desire for distance, and that if the balance were disturbed rapid termination of therapy might easily result.

He continued to experience me as threatening when I tried too soon to talk with him about some aspects of his psychodynamics, and comments on the transference relationship triggered physical anxiety. He often reacted in sessions with skin symptoms (acute and extreme itchiness). I had a feeling that he was extremely frail—"thin skinned" in both senses of the word; I felt as if I were juggling a soap bubble that a gust of wind or a touch at the wrong time would not lift into the air but, rather, cause to burst.

After a period of experiencing me as threatening and aggressively demanding in the transference, my office became a very reliable and structured "cave" for him. He paid attention to the setup and the pictures, as if the room itself were a predictable secure base that he could approach with less anxiety than he could me.

Sometimes he experienced anxious feelings of depersonalization and could hardly speak. He felt that he was standing apart from himself, observing his lacerated and bleeding body, which was in the process of "dissolving, starting with the skin."

However, he eventually stabilized. Long vacations were crisis points. His skin broke out particularly badly just before a 4-week separation. By then it was less difficult to talk to him about his fears of loss, and he said that he did not know how he would tolerate this "eternal vacation." In the second session to last before I left, he asked hesitantly whether perhaps he could take home with him during that time the picture that he always saw from the couch. It was so familiar to him, it belonged to this room and to me, and he would be able to orient himself by looking at it. I was very relieved by this idea and gladly allowed him to take it that day, as he wanted to test it out at home and see if it worked. He was considerably calmer during the next (the last) session. The picture had found a good place in his apartment. He would "hold on to it" in my absence.

This transitional object allowed him to tolerate the vacation hiatus. The picture was a part of a place that he experienced as secure, a part of the space where I practiced, and a part that belonged to me, that he could keep with him. Apparently, he still needed a concrete picture in order to maintain a sense of security in my absence. In view of the avoidant aspects of his attachment, it is understandable that the room where I conduct therapy should be named and internalized as a place of safety more readily than the direct relationship to me, which activated the more ambivalent parts of his attachment.

After 2½ years, Mr. O. and his girlfriend separated. He was no longer willing to accept her desire for closeness at the level she demanded.

At first he had fantasies about taking a long trip. He had never gone on vacation alone. We had spent many hours on this fantasy, and on how the "expedition," which is what he called the planned trip, would unfold. He now felt much more secure, at least in his awareness that he could continue to separate from me and "explore new continents."

Up until now, this idea had remained a fantasy, so I was very surprised when Mr. O. actually began to think concretely about his "expedition." He bought a vehicle that he converted into a sort of camper, whose living section could be uncoupled from the vehicle itself and left behind. This conversion occupied him intensely for weeks. At each session he proudly reported each new bit of progress. His fantasies now concerned the properties that such a camper must have in order to be a stable, safe, and reliable "caregiver." He eventually coined the metaphor "mother-mobile" for this vehicle that he would take with him on his expedition as a secure base. He considered the fact that he could uncouple the "mother part" from the "mobile part," allowing him to explore the region independently, to be a great advantage, both practically and symbolically. He would be able to have his "mother station" with him on the trip as a secure base. At the same time, he could separate from it when he wanted to explore, in the full knowledge that he could seek out the "mother part" again as needed for such things as sleeping and cooking.

Many weeks after he had completed his house/vehicle, he decided, with considerable excitement, to plan a 3-month expedition. I wondered repeatedly to what extent these plans and fantasies represented a form of resistance that would allow him to avoid working through the transference in the here and now after he became more stable. Nevertheless, I did recognize his growing desire for exploration from the security of his base in therapy: in his fantasies at first but then also concretely with the camper.

Finally Mr. O. set off on his expedition. It left me on tenterhooks, wondering whether everything would go well and if he would return safely. He noticed my anxiety at our last meeting, and he comforted me by saying that he would send me postcards from along the way to let me know that he was still alive and also where he happened to be.

In fact I did receive numerous postcards over the next 3 months from places on his itinerary. I was amazed that he was actually exploring new continents and seeming to make his fantasies come true. The trip was not without problems; his mother-mobile left him in the lurch several times and had to be repaired. Luckily, he was able to get help, and thanks to his own mechanical skills he was able to do a number of repairs himself.

I would become uneasy when I didn't receive a postcard from him for a while and then would be relieved when two would arrive at once. I followed his itinerary on a map, and so for those 3 months I was attached to him in my thoughts and emotions.

Three months after his departure, he stood beaming with his "mother-mobile" in front of my office. He arrived punctually at the time he had set before he left. He had a great many experiences to relate. I was happy for him and relieved that he had survived the trip so well.

From that time forward, he entered a phase of separation from me and from his therapy. He was able to think about terminating without troublesome fears or new skin outbreaks.

Upon termination he gave me a picture that he had brought back from his trip. He thought that I should hang it in my office so that I could remember him in his absence—the same way that the picture from my office had helped him to endure separation during my first long vacation.

*Concluding Remarks and Follow-Up*

Mr. O.'s therapy, which lasted 3½ years, at three and sometimes four sessions a week, had led to marked ego stabilization. Building on attachment dynamics, we were able to work through his disorganized attachment relationship to his mother in particular and his difficult relationship with his sister.

At times, I was almost certainly both mother and father to him in the transference. Particularly during the last phase of therapy, when he was planning his trip, it became clear that he wanted to talk to me "man to man" about the expedition. With a foundation of growing attachment security, it became possible for him to realize his desire for individuation and exploration at the concrete as well as the symbolic level. His invention of the mother-mobile allowed him to go long distances from his secure place in therapy for a long period of time, because he was able to take his secure base (in the form of the mother-part) with him.

Although his neurodermatitis was not cured, he had no more acute outbreaks. This in and of itself was a great relief to him. By the end of treatment, he could hold his skin "at bay" with ointments; he had no further need of cortisone cream.

I received a wedding announcement from Mr. O. 2 years later and a short letter from which I concluded that he was making his way in life. He had established himself professionally in a new independent business and according to his reports was being successful.

~

## ATTACHMENT DISORDERS IN ADULTS

Using selected disorders in adults, I will now illustrate how the issue of attachment continues to retain its importance in adult symptomatology. We will find patterns of attachment disorders that are similar in some ways to those described earlier among children and adolescents.

### Symptoms of Anxiety, Panic and Agoraphobia

Bowlby (1973) drew attention to the way symptoms of anxiety, panic, and agoraphobia develop, tracing these back to disturbances in attachment development in childhood. In his studies of agoraphobic patients he found four different family patterns of interaction that he considered to be pathogenic in that they caused the development of attachment disorders in children that left them susceptible later to symptoms of agoraphobia in adulthood. Guidano and Liotti (1985) did a follow-up study based on this hypothesis, and they also found typical familial conflict situations in anxiety patients. The children's needs for autonomy and exploration were inhibited by parental restraints and prohibitions; the parents depicted the world outside the family as dangerous and had convinced the children that they would not be able to withstand its dangers without constant parental protection. Furthermore, the parents had threatened to leave these children on their own if they got into trouble. Such threats were transmitted by various means: punishment, parental battles, suicide threats, emotional withdrawal, actual absence, physical or psychological illness, or even actual death.

*Initial Presentation and Symptoms*

The local neurologist telephones. Mrs. R. is about to be admitted on an emergency basis; she is "terrorizing" not only him and the general practitioner, but the entire family as well. In spite of the announced "emergency" and "terror," Mrs. R., an attractive 29-year-old, comes in for admission a few hours later accompanied by her 3-year-old daughter and her husband. She could not part from the child at home, so she brought her along with her. She can't separate from them even for the intake consultation. She lets her husband describe her symptoms while she herself cries quietly, imparting an impression of childishness and helplessness. I have the feeling that I cannot expect anything from her and that I will have to understand her nonverbal communications.

A very concerned Mr. R. reports that since the death of his wife's mother a year and a half ago Mrs. R. has suffered from a racing heart, irregular pulse, elevated blood pressure, trembling in the knees, fainting spells, and anxieties that may even leave her in a panic-like condition. She has not been able to stay at home alone for several weeks. He and her relatives have been taking care of her, but now his vacation time is all used up, and he doesn't know what to do. Over the past several weeks, Mrs. R. has not allowed her daughter to go to preschool. She calls her family physician or the neurologist several times a day, because she fears that she will "drop dead on the spot from a heart attack." Outpatient treatment, including antidepressants, tranquilizers, and neuroleptics prescribed by the neurologist, have brought no relief. On the contrary: his wife is now brooding about her mother's death even more than before. While she used to take care of her sick father, now she can't even do the basic housekeeping. As he finishes, Mrs. R. says in a low voice, "I want to be free and able to live without fear!"

*Patient History*

Mrs. R. was the youngest of five children from a small country village. She has brothers who are 14, 11, and 5 years older than she; her sister is

7 years older. She was the "princess" in the family, spoiled by everyone. She remembers her mother as good-natured and generous, and herself as a "good and timid child" who clung onto her mother's apron strings. Because of this, it was a great shock for her when her mother suddenly fell from her chair, dead of a heart attack, at the age of 68. She describes her father as being loving, as well, although she did not have a "special relationship" with him. Her parents ran a small farm. They worked hard and had little time for the family. The father, who has been in ill health for a fairly long time, depends on Mrs. R.'s care and support. Now she is tormented by the idea that she might lose him as well; it makes her "crazy," and she feels that she could not survive a second death.

Mrs. R. had refused to go to preschool as a child because she "always wanted to be close" to her mother, who took her along when she did her farm work. Even when she was 8 she clung to her mother when she went down to the cellar to fetch wood. When she was 7, her grandmother, in whose bed she had slept, died suddenly of heart failure. Nobody talked to her about this at the time because "death is taboo in the family." After her grandmother's death, Mrs. R. slept between her parents in their bed, only moving back to her own at age 12, "against my mother's protest" but with her 5-year-older brother's support.

After completing high school, Mrs. R. lived with a female friend in a neighboring village, where she completed her professional training. This separation was not difficult because she was able to spend weekends at home with her parents. Subsequently, she worked for several years in her chosen profession, which was "a lot of fun" for her. She married at the age of 23, and her first daughter, with whom she has a "very close" relationship, was born 2 years later. She sleeps with Mrs. R. in her bed and does not go to preschool because, if she did, "both of us would get panicky and fearful." Previously, the daughter, by her presence alone, had been able to help Mrs. R. contain her anxieties during the day, but for several weeks now neither daughter nor any other relatives and/or acquaintances have been able to accomplish this.

*Consideration of Attachment Dynamics*

Mrs. R. described an idealized and apparently secure attachment to her mother. I suspect, however, that her mother, because of the strain of family and farm, and particularly after her own mother's death, was no longer sufficiently available to her daughter as a secure base, in spite of their spatial and physical closeness. The grandmother, whom Mrs. R. had traumatically lost at the age of 7, may in fact have been the attachment figure who provided real security, but because of family taboos and denials no grief work could be done over her death. From then on Mrs. R. clung even more insistently to her mother—who was probably also grieving, but trying to hide this from the children—acting "well-behaved and timid" so as not to endanger their closeness with aggressive quarreling.

Under these circumstances it is understandable that Mrs. R. did not succeed in becoming less enmeshed with her mother. Her rage and disappointment over this could neither be admitted nor expressed, however, as this would have endangered their relationship. She sought closeness to her mother at night in a search for security and comfort, but I suspect that she herself had to serve as her mother's secure base, because it was only in the face of her mother's protests and against her will that she was finally able to "move out" of the marital bed at the age of 12. Here it becomes clear just how much the mother sought to inhibit the development of autonomy in the patient.

The sudden death of Mrs. R.'s own mother was a traumatic repetition of her grandmother's death. The memory of that loss, never processed or grieved, was reawakened. The patient felt "robbed of all security" and "powerless" because she realized that her attempts to control and "shadow" her mother had failed with her death. The awareness that her father, her secondary attachment figure, could also die put her "into a panic."

With the support of her woman friend, the patient had been able to take some small steps toward individuation when she undertook her professional training; however, her overly close connection to her parents did not loosen.

Through her early marriage the patient was able to establish a symbiotic pattern in her relationship with her husband similar to the one she had had with her mother. However, her husband's changing shifts at work annoyed her, and the nights were a particular "horror." The husband was very sensitive to her needs during the intake consultation, and he showed himself to be caring when he brought her in, but the demands of his own work made it impossible for him to take care of her 24 hours a day. For a while her relationship with her small daughter gave the patient enough security to tolerate her anxieties. But this system had broken down, possibly because of the demands of caring for her father and the thought that she might lose him.

It therefore appeared to me that the patient was repeating her own childhood relationship patterns in the present, creating a constellation in which she, now a mother, urgently needed her own child to protect her from her anxieties. This behavior caused her daughter—as it had caused the patient in childhood—to give up her own desires for exploration and autonomy. The daughter is not allowed to go to preschool and is developing anxieties of her own that threaten to replicate the attachment disorder in the next generation. The basic conflict, both for the patient and for her daughter, might be expressed as follows: "I want to be free to explore the world and go to preschool when I want to. However, I feel that my mother needs me close by. Something could happen to her. In the worst case, she might leave me or die of fear. So, I will stay with her because I need *her* more than preschool. At least when I am home, I can make sure that nothing happens to her. I don't want to tell her how annoyed I am that I have to stay at home because of her; I fear it will make things worse if she feels my anger."

An alternative ready explanation of this patient's psychodynamics might be an unresolved oedipal conflict, which broke out into the open when her mother died and her relationship to her father intensified, perhaps for the first time in her life, because of her daily caregiving duties.

*Therapy and Course*

Mrs. R. adapted relatively quickly to the psychiatric unit. She was a "good" patient, avoiding any conflict with other patients and staff by skillfully accommodating herself to their needs. At first, she wanted to meet with me daily, and in these conversations she initially complained about her heart symptoms, dizziness, and anxieties. She was able to attach to me as a physician who would take care of her physical complaints. However, I reacted to her physical complaints with annoyance; I felt tightly controlled by her symptoms. I recalled that the referring neurologist had talked about how she "terrorized" the family. If she complained about her symptoms, she did not have to talk about her feelings, thereby regulating closeness and distance in our relationship.

After 2 weeks had gone by, she felt physically more stable as long as she was on the unit. Her complaints and anxieties receded into the background. She was able to participate actively in the life of the unit. We were able to negotiate a reduction in sessions to three per week because Mrs. R. was increasingly able to experience both the unit and me as a secure base. Weekend leaves went satisfactorily, although Mrs. R. found it increasingly hard over time to leave home and return to the unit. Although she felt homesick during the week, the thought of being discharged also made her very anxious. She responded with renewed fainting spells and heart palpitations to my attempt to "speed up" her development of autonomy by having her participate in group psychotherapy, and she expressed her own wishes for the first time, requesting continuation of her individual therapy and refusing the "order" to go to group therapy. I was aware of how steadily she sought to establish attachment and contact with me, and to regulate the relationship by intensification of her symptoms. I was surprised when therapy was terminated prematurely after 12 weeks on the husband's urging—he wanted his wife home again. As before, Mrs. R. was very ambivalent about this. She was eventually discharged at her request because I recognized how much she missed her home, surroundings, and family. In addition, I considered a longer separation from her 3-year-old daughter to be detrimental to the child's development.

Mrs. R. wanted to continue to work with me, which I did not consider practical since she lived about an hour's drive away. Instead, I referred her to a closer colleague for outpatient therapy. Six weeks later, Mrs. R. called me again. She reported that she had not been able to find a therapist in her area and that she wanted to continue with me in spite of the distance involved. By then she was somewhat less anxious at home, and she was able to bridge the time between her husband's shifts at work, which she spent alone, "more or less well." But she could not imagine how she would survive the long trip to therapy by herself.

In the end she made a variety of arrangements—at first with her husband and later with a woman friend—who drove her to therapy twice a week. She enjoyed these trips and became increasingly symptom-free because the company made her feel more secure. Still, during the entire first year of therapy, she did not feel stable enough to risk the distance all by herself. Eventually, it became clear that Mrs. R. had found two places of safety: her home environment and the relationship with her husband, and the clinic and her relationship with me. With her husband as "secure driver," she was able to travel the long distance to therapy or go on trips near her home without symptoms. Although before she had been unable to drive to the nearest supermarket alone without feeling dizzy, she was now occasionally able to do this ("with my heart racing") if she prepared herself in advance and could imagine that her husband, a good friend, or I was sitting next to her in the car while she drove. In her fantasy, she was able to "hold onto the driver."

At first, we worked face-to-face; later Mrs. R. lay on the couch. The first few times she tried this, she experienced dizziness—"as if the floor were moving"—and heart palpitations. Only when I pulled my chair next to the couch, so that she could make eye contact with me and reassure herself with my presence, did these symptoms abate.

Grief work over the losses of her grandmother and mother occupied the first phase of therapy. With great effort, Mrs. R. was able to recall scenes: the grandmother's laying out at home, her burial, and Mrs. R.'s parents' "secretiveness." Over time it became clear that the patient's mother "had always been there" but had not really been available emotionally as a secure base. Apparently, Mrs. R.'s mother had taken her daughter into her bed after the grandmother's death in order to feel her daughter's emotional support. But this meant that Mrs. R. had to give up the development of her own individuation and autonomy. Closeness to her mother consisted of Mrs. R.'s "shadowing" her constantly.

Mrs. R. disclosed to me during this initial phase that she was again pregnant. This seemed to her a "wonderful" solution: she could control her abandonment fears by creating a close relationship with her child. She experienced the pregnancy very intensely as a "happy time." Although at first she could not imagine separation from this child at the end of the pregnancy, the subject of the birth began to take on greater importance. She gave birth to a healthy girl. After a short interruption, therapy resumed, and she sometimes left the child in the care of her husband.

After a year of therapy, which Mrs. R. experienced as "a sort of pregnancy" in her emotional development, she was able for the first time to drive to the session alone. In her fantasy, she drove "as if she were on the high seas, from one port to the next." Sometimes she stopped along the way because the distance still seemed "endlessly long," and she didn't think she could tolerate the physical tension. Eventually, however, her car became a place of security as well, her husband having checked it out for "reliability" before she took the wheel. She felt it to be a "safe conveyance" that she could rely on.

In a subsequent phase, Mrs. R.'s relationship with her mother-in-law began to take on greater importance. The anger and disappointment that she felt toward her own mother had been projected onto her mother-in-law, with whom she argued fiercely. The patient was now able to speak, but only hesitantly, about her disappointment in her mother, whom she had always idealized. Memories began to emerge: when she was a small child, the mother had brought her along in a pack basket when she did fieldwork, had set her down somewhere, and left her "to wait forever." Over time, her relationship with her mother-in-law slowly improved, so that Mrs. R. was able to draw her into caring for the children "in an emergency."

Her relationship with her father now became our focus in therapy. The patient realized just how little she had known her father as a child; now she was able to restructure the relationship with him, seeing him not *only* as someone who might die soon.

Over the entire initial phase of our work, Mrs. R. greatly idealized her relationship with me. When sessions ended, and during the separations resulting from vacations and illnesses, Mrs. R.'s symptoms would intensify, and at first she vehemently rejected any attempts to interpret this as an expression of hostile feelings. Only later did it become possible to talk about the rage and disappointment she felt when I was not constantly at her disposal.

This also presented the possibility of working through oedipal transference aspects, which, however, are not the focus of this discussion.

After almost 3 years and approximately 250 hours of treatment, Mrs. R. began, for the first time, to think about terminating therapy. By now she was able to run her household independently, take care of her children, and come to therapy without inordinate anxiety. She tolerated periods of solitude much better. Only occasionally did she now react with anxious irritation when, for example, her husband got home later than expected after working the night shift. A period of intense dreams followed, which depicted leave-taking in all its variations. After working through issues of terminating therapy, Mrs. R. was finally able to say good-bye to me before Christmas, at a time of her own choosing. She called me occasionally after that, just to reassure herself that I could still be found in the same place.

Almost a year later, I received a very anxious call from Mrs. R., who said that she was beginning to suffer from all of the old symptoms again. She realized that this was connected with the fact that her younger daughter would soon be starting preschool, but even though this connection was relatively clear she felt that she might still need my support in handling this separation. I saw the patient for 10 more sessions, in which she focused intently on the relationship with her daughter as a separate individual and the impending year of preschool. Both the trigger and the issues were clear to Mrs. R., but she needed me again as a support to get through this phase. We met over the period when her daughter attended preschool for the first time, and Mrs. R. had to leave her at the school door. She came to therapy for the next few weeks so that she could "really feel sure that everything would be all right." After that, she said good-bye once more, with the understanding that she could call me again in similar difficult situations.

### Concluding Remarks and Follow-Up

This treatment shows that Mrs. R. probably had an insecure-ambivalent attachment to her mother. Although she lived close to her mother, she had hostile feelings toward her, both because of her frustrated desire for attachment and of her inability to experience autonomy and exploration. She had lived through two traumatic situations:

the sudden deaths of her grandmother and her mother. She had not been able to grieve over either loss, and after the death of her mother this finally led to an emotional crisis, which was characterized by psychosomatic symptoms, anxiety, and panic attacks as well as agoraphobic symptoms. These symptoms enabled her to secure the reassuring presence of another person at all times. It became clear that Mrs. R. constantly needed other people as secure bases to stabilize herself emotionally.[6]

The clinic, the psychiatric unit, and the attachment relationship with me represented securities that she could not and did not want to give up after her discharge. This made clear to me how hard it is for such patients to switch from inpatient to outpatient treatment when neither the place nor the secure attachment relationship can be transferred easily to other therapists. If continuing treatment with the same therapist is not possible, patients with anxiety disorders especially require a planned phase-in of the new therapist during the inpatient period.

Mrs. R. was able to rely on me again as an auxiliary secure base when her second daughter began preschool, confronting her with separation. Although Mrs. R. was able to reflect on this problem by herself, she still needed me for emotional support so that she could allow her daughter to go through the separation process. At that time I was doubtful about whether the treatment had succeeded, since the patient still needed to call me frequently. I therefore focused on the resolution of transference issues.

Over the past several years I occasionally received Christmas cards from this former patient, who enclosed greetings and some brief thoughts. I read these cards with mixed feelings because I wasn't sure how to interpret them. Ten years later, I learned from the patient that she was completely immersed in her former profession and that she was now looking forward to her adolescent daughter's increasing autonomy. It turned out that the Christmas cards had been inspired by her memories of terminating therapy before Christmas and recalling our good-bye during the beginning of Advent. Thus, she had intended the cards as a brief message that things were going well for her.

## Depressive Symptoms

*Initial Presentation and Symptoms*

Mrs. W., age 55, comes to the clinic accompanied by her husband. Her family physician has ordered her admission because she has become progressively more depressed over the preceding several weeks. Now she clings to her husband's arm, and he accompanies her into the interview room; she insists that he come along and also that he report the history of her acute symptoms. Mrs. W. sits hunched and dejected in her chair; she is stiff, expressionless, and almost motionless. The husband, clearly moved, reports that his wife has changed completely over the past several months. Once she had been active and energetic, taking care of the house and children. Now she spends hours lying in bed in the morning and can't do the housekeeping; things are piled up all around. She nods and agrees, tears rolling down her face. Talking about herself, or everything else for that matter, has become too much for her. She is very depressed about the change. Previously she had been known as an excellent housewife and mother who easily kept house and garden under control. Some days she finds it hard even to get dressed, let alone to clean, tidy up, or bake a cake. Treatment with antidepressants has not been very successful; over the past 2 weeks things have actually gotten considerably worse. When I ask about it, Mrs. W. reports that she occasionally thinks about suicide. She feels that she can't go on this way; she would rather be dead, so ashamed does she feel, and so guilty about her husband and children. A person who has sunk so low, she says, has no right to live.

*Patient History*

Mrs. W. was the oldest of four children. Her two sisters are 3 and 8 years younger, and her brother 5 years younger, than she. Even when she was very young she supported her mother in the house and in raising the children. Everyone considered her diligent, purposeful, and friendly. She met her present husband when she was 19, and married at 21—as soon as she came of age—so that she could "finally get out of the house."

Her greatest wish had always been to have a large family like the one she had grown up in, and she had three children, two daughters and a son, at intervals of 2 years. She had felt completely fulfilled and happy raising the children, building the house, taking care of the garden, and supporting her husband in his career. It had been a lot of work, but these had been the happiest years of her life. Her husband was secure and well-respected in his work, and all of her children had been successful as well. She had been very affected by the departure of the children when they moved away to study or to work.

This depression was triggered by her son's announcement that he wanted to get married soon, at the age of 22. This was completely incomprehensible to her. He was in the middle of his studies, and she felt that he should complete his professional training and achieve financial security before starting a family. Mrs. W. brooded about this day and night, but she could not convince her son, and she wondered what she had done wrong. Thank God, her daughters were ambitious and worked hard, and they visited her more often, now that she was ill. This had become a necessity, if only because she needed help with the housework and the large garden. Previously, though, she had always been able to cope with these herself.

## Consideration of Attachment Dynamics

It is probable that this patient had been given the role of mothering her siblings early in life and had had to serve as their attachment figure. Presumably, her own desire and need for attachment security was not adequately satisfied, as she was forced to accept too much responsibility at too early an age, and to curtail her own desire for exploration. This is the pattern she repeated in her own marriage. Her deliberately managed early home-leaving at the age of 21 can be interpreted as a reaction formation. In order to be no longer burdened with the responsibility for her siblings and her family of origin, she tried to free herself of her role as attachment figure. She could only do this by marrying early, and against her father's will.

Mrs. W. recalls her role as mother and housewife as having been very satisfying and fulfilling. There was much closeness between her and her children. From the attachment and exploration viewpoint, she felt that she served her children both as a "safe haven" and as a secure base. The depressive crisis and the inability to deal with the children's autonomy had only begun to emerge as they began to develop in age-appropriate ways away from the family.

The triggering event that Mrs. W. describes, the planned early marriage of her youngest son, re-evokes the other attachment losses that Mrs. W. has suffered, and which she cannot work through because she can accept neither her own nor her children's individuation. These difficulties now come to a head with her children's developing independence. The depression intensifies her clinginess to her daughters. Her husband often stays home, thereby neglecting his own professional obligations. He brings her to the clinic and visits her often. In general, her attachment relationships become more anxious, but at the same time Mrs. W. feels herself unloved and shoved into the clinic; she reproaches her family because inpatient admission represents a separation from them that causes her a great deal of anxiety and that she is unable to process emotionally. The decision to admit her was made because of the increasing danger of suicide, but it had also led to an intense preoccupation with attachment. On the one hand, inpatient admission had intensified the unconscious desire for contact with the family even though Mrs. W. consciously felt "lonely and abandoned." On the other hand, treatment in the clinic made possible a physical separation from the primary family and thus fulfilled the patient's desire for autonomy and individuation.

### Therapy and Course

Mrs. W. presented as endogenously depressed. She cannot understand or reconstruct why she has become so depressed. To the outside observer, there is a definable trigger: namely, the son's impending marriage. But the patient herself cannot reconstruct the conflict around this or understand why the impending separation from her son would trigger depression of such severity. For this reason she is not open to explanations that center on her conflict with her son. She feels very bad, but without knowing why. As far she is concerned, this terrible illness has come out of the blue, and she just hopes that it will abate again. She views it as the kind of stroke of fate that one simply has to survive.

In accordance with our understanding of her attachment dynamics, Mrs. W. was assigned a "reference person" or caregiver on the unit whose role it was to be available to serve as her primary advocate. All family contacts, their duration and frequency, and all leaves (initially in the company of the caregiver) were agreed to in direct discussions between Mrs. W. and this designated individual, and in consultation with the therapist. Initially, these contacts took place at 30-minute intervals and lasted no more than 5 minutes each.

It turned out that the patient's suicidal tendencies were more concrete, and therefore also more serious, than had appeared on admission, so she was to contact her designated caregiver (or a substitute if the caregiver was not on duty) every half hour during the first several days. If the designated caregiver left the unit, responsibility for the patient was always transferred to a substitute. That is, a great deal of attention was paid to relationship constancy and closeness, and as a result Mrs. W. knew that there was always a specific caregiver assigned directly to her. If she failed to report at the specified time, the caregiver would look for her to see how she was doing and to reestablish the attachment relationship from his side. This resulted in a very intense relationship. After 2 weeks the severity of Mrs. W.'s depression began to decrease without changes having been made in her antidepressive treatment (which on admission seemed to have been adequate). Husband and children were regularly mobilized to provide care and companionship; Mrs. W. could telephone family members regularly and go for walks with them. Weekend leaves, however, were not possible at first because of the considerable suicide risk. Mrs. W. found it difficult to make arrangements for the entire weekend for fear of her suicidal tendencies. She did not know whether attachment relationships with her own family, which, after all, were going through major changes, would give her as much security and stability as the supportive milieu and "holding" relationships available to her on the unit.

In the individual sessions we focused primarily on Mrs. W.'s symptoms. I tried to accept her complaining and reproachful attitude toward her children and husband, by whom she felt abandoned because she thought they visited much too infrequently. My attempts to address her need to feel cared for were initially rejected with a shrug. She came regularly to individual sessions, which at first took place thrice weekly, but this was not enough for her. At the end of the hour she had a difficult time separating and would begin to complain about sleep disorders and her lack of motivation while we were saying good-bye.

After 2 weeks she also began to participate in group psychotherapy, which consisted of a combination of movement therapy and verbal processing of what she experienced there. The group also allowed her to identify with other patients and become less dependent on the staff and myself. Mrs. W. soon felt accepted in the group, which included other women of her age with similar depressive symptoms. In addition, the group included young patients who were dealing with postadolescent autonomy, and because of this the issues of separation and attachment began to be addressed more frequently. As a result, Mrs. W., whose symptoms were slowly improving, was also able to grapple with the issue of autonomy in individual therapy. The young people in the group reminded her of her own children who "were now growing up and leaving home."

Over the course of treatment, she became able to understand the extent to which she had satisfied her own unfulfilled early attachment needs by creating close attachment relationships with her children. Relationships outside the family were not so important to her, because her need for attachment was fully satisfied by her emotional closeness to her children and to her husband. She said that she did not know what she would do with herself without the children and her household, because autonomy, exploration, and the concept of a life of her own still seemed very foreign to her.

She was introduced to new possibilities for creative activity in occupational therapy on the unit. She developed a passion for painting on silk. For the first time in her life, she had time to pursue interests and hobbies that she had never considered while she was involved with her family. On weekend leaves she was able to discover and create a "new partnership" with her husband that did not include the children. Over time she began to enjoy hiking and bicycling on the weekend, and she came to see that life with her husband "could be meaningful in old age" too.

By then, her son's relationship with the girlfriend he had originally intended to marry had broken up. Mrs. W. was very relieved, even though she now understood that her son's marriage plans had been only a part of her problem. It looked as if the children, too, could now work on their own autonomy, encouraged by their mother's successful processing of individuation issues.

### Concluding Remarks and Follow-Up

Mrs. W. developed a very close relationship with another female patient, whom she continued to see after discharge. Outpatient treatment continued at longer intervals; the frequency of sessions was left up to the patient herself. She came in for outpatient sessions about once or twice a month. As she no longer had to take her family and children into consideration, these sessions usually revolved around her newly gained autonomy and the possibilities that her new hobbies presented.

Mrs. W.'s admission occurred as the result of a severe depressive crisis resembling an endogenous depression with suicidal tendencies. It was not possible at first to work with her conflicts, as she had no access to them. Both the setting on the unit and the very tight caregiving regimen used there were designed to fulfill Mrs. W.'s need for attachment security. As a result of this developing base, Mrs. W. was able to work through her fears of separation and pursue new ways of exerting autonomy. Outpatient follow-up treatment showed that Mrs. W. was becoming more self-reliant and becoming less needful of the constant emotional presence of her husband and children. The use of antidepressants alone would almost certainly not have adequately addressed the patient's need for attachment and exploration, let alone satisfied that need.

The fear that inpatient hospitalization might deepen a depression further is not justified if carefully thought out and if structured supportive contact is made available. Mrs. W.'s ego functions were stabilized by the structuring of her relationship with her primary caregiver and by clearly defined beginning and end points. With the increasingly stable secure base that she developed during her inpatient treatment, Mrs. W. dared to grieve both her separation from, and the restructuring of, her

family—both her family of origin and her present family—and begin
the process of exploration and individuation.

## Narcissistic Symptoms

I have already discussed the link between the development of self-
esteem and attachment in the theoretical section. The development of a
secure attachment based on an attachment figure's sensitive caregiving
is an important prerequisite for the construction of a stable sense of self-
worth.

### Initial Presentation and Symptoms

A handsome and well-dressed middle-aged man in suit and tie comes to
an initial consultation that he had sought because of difficulties working and concentrating. His youthful and dynamic appearance is somewhat belied by his graying temples. Mr. Z. dominates the conversation
from the outset and asks precise questions. In the countertransference, I
feel like a student at an oral exam. I get the impression that Mr. Z. is
becoming increasingly anxious about the possibility that I might participate actively by asking him questions, or that some sort of relationship
might actually develop between us. Mr. Z. has come to me for concrete
suggestions—or, better, for an educational program—that will enable
him to get his concentration problem under control. He is irritated
when I tell him that I have no such program, especially when I don't
know much about the onset or cause of his concentration disorder.
Eventually, he tells me hesitantly and in bits and pieces: it all began 6
months ago when his wife suddenly left him.

### Patient History

Mr. Z. is the oldest of three sons, with brothers 1 and 4 years younger
than he. He had always been "the big guy," the successful son loved by
his parents for his accomplishments, leadership, and commitment. He
idealized and spoke with great admiration of his father, whom he had
begun to help with his business at an early age. For his whole life he
had had very rivalrous relationships with his brothers in which things

had generally gone his way. As the first-born and crown prince of the family, he had always been helped and supported. He was very well liked in preschool. He was a favorite of his teachers in school because of his high achievement, and he completed his studies with flying colors. After a number of affairs and while still a student, he met his present wife, and they were soon married. She is a very attractive woman, and, as far as he is concerned, she was made for the role of mother to his children. The couple had a daughter and a son, but Mr. Z. does not describe a particularly close relationship. At the time of the children's birth he had been very much involved in work and had only been able to spend a few hours a week at home. Housekeeping and child-rearing were his wife's "department." His children were as successful as he was and had completed their studies with distinction. Mr. Z. appears very proud of his children as he relates this. When I ask him about his relationship to his wife, he shrugs his shoulders. Everything was going OK, and so he can't understand why she suddenly packed her bags 6 months ago and moved out. She told him that she finally wanted a life of her own, to be free and independent, and to enjoy life. She had never lacked for anything in the marriage, and they never worried about financial matters. He says that he has no problems with relationships and that he gets along with everybody. He is valued for his diplomacy in business matters, women like him, and many people envy his success. He has never had any real problems before. Over the past several weeks, however, his sleep and concentration difficulties have become so severe that he now needs concrete help. When asked about friends and other important people, Mr. Z. says that he has a lot of friends—business friends and sports friends; he is a social person. However, I sense that there has never actually been a person in his life with whom he has had a genuine emotional relationship.

## Consideration of Attachment Dynamics

I suspect that Mr. Z.'s childhood attachment relationship to his mother and father had been rather avoidant. Evidently, achievement and success were highly prized in the family, and attachment and relationship were exclusively defined around them. Obviously, Mr. Z.'s achievements and success were in line with his parents' ideal. In addition, he idealized his parents, especially his very successful father, because of their achievements, and they served as role models for him. His internal working model may be telling him that close relationships can be established and maintained through achievement and success. However, a genuine emotional attachment in which Mr. Z. could feel "at home" was something that he had not yet experienced. He describes his relationship to his own children and to his wife as functional and well organized, but without emotional involvement or perceptible attachment. In the same way, he tries to keep me at a distance, to control me and functionalize our relationship to the extent that I am there merely to serve as advisor for the educational program he desires. Evidently, this is a typical dismissing, functionally-oriented relational strategy; Mr. Z. employs it successfully in business, but it gives him no way to enter emotionally into the psychotherapeutic relationship, or even into a close relationship with his family.

Against this backdrop, it is understandable that his wife, having completed her child-rearing duties, left him once the children had finished school. Even given this attachment-avoidant background, his family and his relationship with his wife evidently provide him a certain amount of security and help orient him. He is very pained by her departure, and is so emotionally unnerved that he reacts with psychosomatic sleep and concentration disorders that can also be understood as depression. Even though his relationship with his wife had not been close, consonant with his avoidant attachment pattern, her departure is nevertheless a loss, which points to his actual attachment desire and need.

From a self psychological perspective, one could say that Mr. Z. has a severe narcissistic disorder and that he has been able compensate for it up until now by achievement and business successes and by the way he arranged his family life. Mr. Z. had not been confronted with deficits in the development of his self-worth, or with other narcissistic injuries, because up until now his life had consisted only of successes. He had been successful in maintaining the grandiose fantasies that his parents had nourished since his childhood. Now, bothered by sleep and concentration problems, he fears that the professional success that he has had to date could evaporate. With justification, he feels insecure and anxious that the narcissistic edifice he has built could collapse.

*Therapy and Course*

Initially, I was skeptical about offering Mr. Z. therapy based on attachment dynamics, because it became clear during the initial consultation how greatly he had organized his life around avoidant attachment and narcissistic success. He was looking for a therapeutic recipe, a program to help him get a handle on his sleep and concentration disorders. Perhaps this could be better accomplished with behavioral therapy, and without confronting him unduly with his attachment anxieties. On the other hand, this depressive crisis had been triggered by the separation from his wife; he felt wounded and insecure because his wife no longer served as a secure haven for his existent attachment needs, however distancing these might be.

With these aspects of attachment dynamics in mind, I decided on a treatment strategy aimed at Mr. Z.'s unconscious and hidden attachment desires. I knew full well how difficult it is to strike a balance between making attachment available while at the same time not offering too much, given the wariness of close relationships that patients with avoidant attachment problems experience. It took us a long time to find a date for our second appointment in Mr. Z.'s busy schedule. Apart from his actual work overload, this interaction also revealed his fear of attachment. I patiently helped him look for a date for our next appointment, which was to be 4 weeks after the first one. Mr. Z. was not at all bothered by the long interval; this was precisely the sort of distance that offered him security, while at the same time not threatening his attachment dynamics. Over the course of therapy, Mr. Z.'s calendar, that is, his avoidant orientation, determined closeness, and therefore also the frequency of treatment.

During the initial phase our dialogues revolved around his sleep and concentration disorders, the demands of his job, and the success that he achieved nonetheless. Following the pattern he had adopted vis-à-vis his parents, he wanted me to admire him as a successful patient. He made a great effort to "achieve success" with his symptoms; perhaps he might even become my star patient. Evidently this was the only way he could imagine being seen, liked, and sheltered in an attachment relationship. During this phase I did not formulate any interpretations of his attachment dynamics. Instead, I decided to go along with Mr. Z.'s approach to relationships; he was operating within an attachment pattern that was comfortable for him and that let him make contact with me and continue our dialogue without having to run away out of his fear of closeness. A tighter setting would certainly have increased his attachment anxieties to the point where he would have acted out more or even terminated therapy.

After having just seen his wife again at the divorce negotiations, Mr. Z. was very upset when he arrived at his next session. She had been cold and distant toward him and only wanted to talk about financial matters. He, however, still liked her very much and would have liked to go out with her in the evening, a notion that she absolutely rejected. He experienced this continued rebuff and rejection—her "coldness"—as brutal. He couldn't understand the change that had come over her. This was the thanks he got for his years of financial support; he had built a fortune, and it had provided security for her and the family. He feared that she now wanted only to bleed him dry; she accused him of having been interested only in material things and said that he had never really been interested in her. This upset him deeply; after all, he had taken care of the family loyally for all these years. Perhaps he had been unable to give her the sense of closeness and protection that she had hoped for in the relationship. The children were evidently on her side, which further threatened and upset him. He was forced to recognize that he was very isolated and alone.

This event gave me my first opportunity to talk about his desire for relationship and his longing for closeness, protection, and belonging. For the first time, at this very turbulent session, he was able to hear it. I very carefully chose how much to talk about these desires; I was extremely careful to avoid intensifying the depressive crisis, which would have occurred had he suddenly felt for the first time the full weight of his feeling of aloneness and his desire for attachment. In addition, he could not afford to be incapacitated at work. However, I also felt that he was very relieved to be able to talk about these experiences and feelings with another person. From then on, our relationship in therapy deepened, even though the frequency of the sessions varied greatly. By then, Mr. Z. was able to make room in his calendar for therapy as if it were any other meeting; in other words, he gave me a place in his life. This also meant that he now gave the therapeutic relationship value and room in his otherwise functionally organized life.

Mr. Z. remained in therapy for a total of more than 3 years. During this time I accompanied him in his grief work around the separation and divorce from his wife. Over the course of this grief work, and as a result of our relationship, Mr. Z. became increasingly aware of his own desire and need for protection, security, and belonging. He experienced painful feelings of grief and rage that were almost too much to bear. He feared that an emotional breakdown would lead to unemployment, that he would lose his job, that he would fail, be rejected, and eventually stand "before the abyss," in terms of family and profession both. This enormous fear could only be grasped and contained because he was able to use the therapist as a secure base. Without this, he would not have been able to explore his need for attachment. During our last year, it was very painful for him to feel and increasingly recognize that his needs as a child had not been met by his parents. He came to feel abused by his parents, who had cast him in the role of achiever and praised him as the crown prince while failing to satisfy his real needs. With horror he recognized that he had raised his children according to the same principle, namely, that achievement and success where the most important things in life. He became painfully aware that, to be truly successful, achievement must be anchored in a secure foundation of attachment dynamics.

Although Mr. Z. initially tried to "make up for" the loss of his wife through short-term acquaintances and relationships, by the end of therapy he was able to find a new partner, and he entered into a relationship with her that evidently had more closeness and emotion than he had experienced to date.

*Concluding Remarks and Follow-Up*

Mr. Z. became vulnerable as a result of his separation from his wife. In therapy he was able to work through the acute depressive crisis. He was able to feel his early desires and deficits in the context of the attachment security developed in therapy. He was eventually able to integrate these as components of his new emotional security. This gave him the security he needed to enter into a new partnership built on an emotionally more secure foundation. From a therapeutic perspective, it was very important to recognize his desire for closeness at the outset, while at the same time taking into account his avoidant and very dismissing interactional pattern. It was crucial not to destabilize this pattern by forcing attachment and relationship on him, thereby provoking termination. This care alone made it possible for Mr. Z. to enter into a closer relationship and allow his unconscious desires and needs, which had not been met in childhood, to express themselves.

This therapeutic procedure reminds me of the technique developed by Kohut in his self psychology. However, even though the empathic therapeutic stance demanded by Kohut does intersect with an attachment-oriented technique, the primary focus on attachment dynamics differs from Kohut's approach.

## Borderline Symptoms

*Initial Presentation and Symptoms*

Ms. N.'s mother calls to make an outpatient appointment for her 21-year-old daughter. She is not sure whether her daughter will agree to therapy or even to an initial consultation; she is an adult and can't be compelled. The mother begins a long and pressured monologue over the phone. I am not sure precisely who needs relief and help. Eventually the daughter does comes in for an initial consultation, accompanied by her mother, who is visibly irritated when I introduce myself in the waiting room and tell her that I want first to speak to her daughter alone. The daughter seems to interpret this as a sign of respect, however, and, contrary to her mother's expectations, she sits down willingly for our initial meeting. She looks critical and skeptical as well as expectant and demanding, and I sense that she will test me. Ms. N. is youthfully dressed, and she wears a good deal of makeup; there is a pronounced (and lingering) scent of perfume in the room. Ms. N. remains silent; she wants me to ask questions. A dialogue develops about whether she wants to talk or remain silent, or whether she wants me to guess which. We are entangled after only a few minutes, and I still have no idea about why she is there. I have the feeling that there is no escape, no possibility of evading this entanglement. I see what would classically be viewed as Ms. N.'s "acting out" as an attempt to make some sort of connection with me in the face of a fear that I will deceive her.

We spend a good deal of time at the end of the hour on whether or not Ms. N. will come back. It is important to her that I talk only with her and not with her mother. We schedule another appointment, although Ms. N. leaves open whether she will actually come.

At the end of the consultation, the mother urgently wants to talk to me alone. I decline, pointing out that her daughter is an adult and that this is her therapy. I raise the possibility to the mother that she could look for a therapist for herself; she is very annoyed by this. Later that same day, she calls and tries to describe part of her daughter's history; again I decline to listen, pointing out that this is the daughter's therapy and that she herself might want to begin therapy elsewhere. The way in which the mother crosses boundaries is diagnostically significant, because it mirrors the mother's competition with the daughter and demonstrates how she tries to preempt the daughter's therapeutic relationship to me.

Ms. N. is 20 minutes late for our second session. She is still ambivalent about coming and doesn't expect much from therapy; perhaps it would be better if she saw a female therapist. I feel that she is struggling: she is soliciting a relationship with me and at the same time signaling rejection and refusal. The next day, Ms. N. calls and says that she urgently needs an appointment—otherwise something terrible will happen. I sense her anxiety, and against my usual principle of maintaining clarity and structure in the therapy setting I schedule an appointment. This time, Ms. N., extremely tense, is in the waiting room 15 minutes early. She has had a violent argument with her mother, who is opposed to my treating Ms. N. because I had refused to talk to her. The patient wants to come to me for therapy, but I have to promise not to accept her mother as a patient as well.

Later I learned that Ms. N. has had terrible arguments with her parents, especially with her mother, for many years. At times the arguments have become physical. In their aftermath Ms. N. often would feel depressed, as if her mother had "steamrollered" her. She was often so

full of rage that she didn't know what to do next. She has attempted suicide four times already by various means: slitting her wrists, taking
pills, and lying down in the forest drunk, after having run away. Sometimes she fantasizes about killing herself or her mother.

### Patient History

Ms. N. is her parents' only child. She was an "accident." Her mother was
only 17 when she became pregnant and married without her parents'
consent. Ms. N.'s father, whom she describes as very authoritarian because he "forbids any freedom," is very different from her mother. Her
mother vacillates; on the one hand she spoils and secretly supports her
daughter, and on the other she gives in to the father's decisions and
opinions. Mother and daughter often unite against the father and together overturn his authoritarian orders. But when the father discovers
his daughter's "misdeeds," the mother does not back her up, but attacks
her, leaving her open to her father's full rage. She experiences this as
"betrayal," and thinks about running away and killing herself. There is
also constant stress at school. Ms. N. is a mediocre, even poor, student,
and whether she will actually complete school or not is unclear. Her
mother has taken care of Ms. N. all her life, but at the same time has
constantly accused her of having "messed up" her (the mother's) life by
having been born in the first place. The patient's history comes out in
such bits and pieces that it is hard to reconstruct it; my task is to construct an image of her history from the puzzle pieces.

### Consideration of Attachment Dynamics

Ms. N. was the product of an unwanted conception and birth. It is likely
that the mother's attitude toward her was highly ambivalent from the
beginning. The pregnancy enabled her mother to leave her parents and
marry Ms. N.'s father. Evidently Ms. N. served as an emotional support
for her mother, but at the same time, Ms. N. constantly experienced her
mother as "stabbing her in the back" when she "caved in" to her father's
authoritarian demands. As a result, the patient felt betrayed by her
mother, and left to fend for herself. She could never tell whether or not

her mother's emotional support was going to be dependable. She had a backlog of experience that told her that she could not rely on her mother, especially when the father exerted pressure. Her close emotional attachment to her mother, on the one hand, and her feelings of having been betrayed by her, on the other, led to an attachment pattern that suggests "entanglement" with aspects of disorganization. Ms. N. demonstrated her ambivalence in the way she structured our initial consultation. She sought closeness, but at the same time was very distressed by the possibility that I might betray her to her mother. Only when I separated the two was Ms. N. able to enter into the therapeutic relationship. However, her mother's acting out exposed her to a great deal of unpleasantness as the mother, upset by my rebuff, attempted to boycott therapy. There was no chance whatsoever that the mother would seek out therapy for herself, given her own disorder.

The patient was still very entangled in her attachment to her father and mother. She had not been able to develop a healthy balance of attachment and autonomy. Ms. N. fought with herself about how to control the aggressive feelings that resulted from her disappointments, her mother's boundary transgressions, and her father's authoritarian attitudes. To Ms. N., the only way out consisted of running away, acts of aggression against herself, or fantasies of destroying her mother.

The preoccupied or entangled attachment pattern that she lived out with her mother established itself relatively quickly toward me during our initial consultation. It was necessary to create a setting clearly structured enough to impart to her a sense of security. But her acting out had also to be taken into account (for example, her emergency phone call) because it was an expression of the patient's attachment disorder; I feared that the patient might terminate therapy if she found me unwilling to serve as an attachment figure in such situations.

From the perspective of classical psychodynamics, all the early defense mechanisms, such as splitting, are apparent. Ms. N. splits her mother into a distinctly caring, even overcaring, good mother, and a bad mother who betrays her and exposes her to her father. From an object relations theory point of view, Ms. N. has not yet developed self or object constancy.

*Therapy and Course*

At first Ms. N. constantly questioned both the setting and the structure of therapy; she forgot or skipped appointments, demanded "urgent appointments" over the phone, or arrived too early or too late. It was very difficult to maintain the necessary structure and constancy while at the same time reacting flexibly enough to take Ms. N.'s attachment needs into account, so that she would not terminate therapy. I did not view her acting out only as resistance. From an attachment perspective, it is an expression of her entangled attachment to her mother, which is now reproduced in the therapeutic relationship.

Over the course of the first year of therapy, Ms. N. "split" the therapist into the one who gave her attachment security and the one who rejected and failed her. Eventually, she was able to understand that ending the session at the end of the hour and observing rules were not an expression of "malevolence and arbitrariness," but a sign of a committed and predictable relationship. As a child, Ms. N. had never known predictability in her relationship with her mother; she had no protection from her mother's arbitrarily changing attachment stances. Weekends, and especially my vacations, were initially reasons for Ms. N. to feel that I was unreliable, uninterested in her, and, finally, rejecting. She believed that she was supposed to function as I expected, and then to come to therapy sessions whenever I happened to have time for her. At the same time, the rush appointments that I made for her, which took place in the structured setting of my office but outside the schedule that we had agreed to, constituted "proof" that she could depend on me as a therapist. In the past, from a classical therapeutic perspective, I would have seen such a procedure as a collusion in her acting out. From my current perspective, however, I now see it as helpful to discuss with the patient the attachment dynamics of this repetitive "acting out," which express specific hopes and desires for the presence and constancy of the attachment figure.

It took about a year for Ms. N. to feel sufficient attachment security in therapy to allow therapy to enter calmer waters. Treatment revolved completely around resolving her entanglement with her mother and creating boundaries with her father. It was very hard during that time not to fall into transference constellations that mirrored her dealings with her parents, that is, oscillating between overcaring and rejection or creating authoritarian structures that made flexible reaction impossible.

Only over the course of the second year of therapy did it become increasingly possible to talk to Ms. N. about her arguments with her parents. By now, she was able to look at these alternating and inconsistent interactions in a more differentiated way, and to take a clearer and more structured stance toward her mother. She also dared to set clearer boundaries for herself in relation to her father, and to stop submitting to his authoritarian demands. Previously, Ms. N.'s circle of friends had been a constantly changing group of chaotic relationships; now, she found a stable place with a group of people who accepted and valued her. She no longer had to exclude herself from a group by acting out before they excluded her.

Toward the end of therapy, Ms. N. had gained sufficient security to enable her to enter into a stable couple relationship with a partner. She thought of therapy as no longer important, wanting to spend her time with her partner and her group of friends.

*Concluding Remarks*

At the beginning of therapy, Ms. N. reenacted in the transference her entangled attachment relationship with her mother. Her acting out in the form of self-directed aggressive actions and suicide attempts indicates that Ms. N. had to fight against the experience of archaic and disorganizing rage. As a result of the security and stability that she gained in the therapeutic relationship, she became able to feel her own attachment security and constancy; she could now tolerate separation from the therapist, and no longer needed to react by acting out and splitting. To this extent, this relationship represented a corrective emotional experience, a new beginning.

From an object relations perspective, it could be said that the patient experienced growing self- and object constancy, corresponding to a secure state of mind with respect to attachment. As a result, Ms. N. was able to let go of the therapeutic relationship and enter into age-appropriate relationships. Perhaps more intensive working through of the patient's archaic destructive and aggressive fantasies might have been appropriate. In therapy, these fantasies were interpreted as an emotional reaction to her frustrated need for attachment. Over the course of treatment, the patient felt sufficiently supported to allow her to look at her self-destructive and other destructive fantasies more clearly without reliving them.

## Psychotic Symptoms

*Initial Presentation and Symptoms*

A 19-year-old is referred by his family physician for an "addiction to computer games," and comes to the initial interview with his mother. Once his mother has left the room, he reports that all of his friends are envious of him because of his computer expertise. It is true that he often plays for hours at a time, but this is necessary to keep in shape and to train. In any case, he has everything under control. He goes on to divulge that he radiates a force that penetrates the computer monitor and affects the combat ability of his fighter jets. He can foresee the outcome of combat; in fact, he has special sensitivity to such radiating forces. At the end of our initial dialogue, he acknowledges that I have a "good force," and so he is willing to come for another session. His manner is conspiratorial and controlling; he looks at me with a sharp, piercing gaze, as though he wants to penetrate and ascertain my thoughts.

*Patient History*

In the course of subsequent dialogues I learn that O. is the youngest of three children. His two older siblings are independent and no longer live with their parents. O. became interested in electronics at a very early age because his father worked in the field. The father especially was very pleased about this and introduced him to computers and computer technology, so O.'s interest in these things was not seen as particularly noteworthy. But over the past 4 months his mother had noticed that her son often got up at night and sat in front of the computer playing games and uttering magic formulas to affect the outcome. At such times it was impossible to interrupt him. Often he sat in front of the computer all night long as if in a trance, and during these times he was inaccessible to his parents. Lately he had been saying that his magic powers gave him control over the end of the world.

There had been some strident arguments between father and son when his father had confronted him about his strange electronic theories. O. stated that his father understood nothing about modern electronics, but that he himself can "upload my thoughts to the Internet."

Early on, O.'s mother had introduced him to her very strict faith, in which spiritual thoughts played a great role. For many years, religion facilitated a close attachment relationship between mother and son. At adolescence, however, O. created an age-appropriate boundary between himself and his mother, and no longer accompanied her to religious services. Instead, he spent hours immersing himself in his father's technology.

Over the past few weeks, he had begun to fail in school—surely the result of his psychotic thinking. A very intelligent young man, he still attended classes regularly, and there were phases when he was quite capable of following the lessons. At night, however, he sat in front of his computer completely immersed in his psychotic world.

### Consideration of Attachment Dynamics

Presumably, their common spirituality had led to a close tie between O. and his mother from childhood. In early adolescence, when he was creating boundaries between them, he turned to his father's technology. This facilitated greater independence from his mother, but produced an equally enmeshed attachment to his father. The psychotic symptoms—which included the belief that he was a wizard of the force, who had magic powers over the computer and could affect and change the world—may be interpreted in an attachment context as a simultaneous attempt to maintain his attachment to the mother and her spirituality and to the father and his electronics at the same time. The psychotic symptoms may thus be seen as an attempt to free himself from his very enmeshed relationship with his parents and to discover a world independent of them, and belonging only to him. Only he knew his way around this world, and he could explore his own powers within it. Neither his mother nor his father showed much sensitivity as attachment figures. O. had been used, or abused, by both of them in their own interests. Neither parent sufficiently responded to his age-appropriate needs for attachment and exploration. As a result, he found himself in a dilemma: as long as he maintained a close attachment relationship to his mother, which was based on spirituality, he was her prisoner, and separated from his father. To the extent that he turned radically away from his mother and immersed himself in his father's electronics, he was a prisoner of his father's conception of the world, but then he was separated from his mother. The formation of his delusional symptoms about his power of radiation allowed him an independent perspective; at the same time he maintained constant contact with his parents by way of the ubiquitous force that only he could control. In his omnipotence he was able to control closeness and distance as well as the frequency and intensity of the "radiation" relationship and attachment. This enabled him to maintain autonomy without having to give up his relationship with both parents, although at the cost of delusional symptoms. When he sat in front of his computer at night, he was attached not only to his sleeping parents by means of his potent radiation but to all people worldwide. He could not do without the computer games because the moment he turned them off, he feared that he would become separated from the rest of humanity and be left alone. In other words, his constant addictive game playing also prevented him from feeling lonely and alone.

## Therapy and Course

Both O. and his parents rejected inpatient treatment and/or medication. Neither parents nor son could imagine the separation implied by inpatient admission. This fact alone demonstrated how closely both parents, for their own purposes, were entangled with the boy; they both needed him for their own emotional stability. Because O. had read that one can become dependent on a therapist, his attitude toward therapy was very skeptical at first, and under no circumstances would he agree to more than once a week. Only later, when the therapeutic attachment relationship had stabilized, could the frequency be increased to twice weekly

without causing him great anxiety. I was very skeptical whether such in-
frequent sessions could have any effect, given the severity of his symptoms. But I had no apparent choice but to adapt to the intensity of the
relationship and attachment that O. permitted, and to allow myself to
be guided by him.

At first O. was distrustful and hesitant about inviting me into his delusional world and telling me more about it. I learned only sporadically at
first about his fantasies, which over time revealed themselves as a complex delusional structure. Even without an Internet connection, his radiation force allowed him to be in contact with the entire world. I interpreted
this grandiose expansion of attachment and connection as a sign of loss of
emotional attachment and of secure support in his relationships with his
parents, and simultaneously as an attempt to individuate.

Relatively soon O. came to believe that he was connected to me
telepathically and could read my thoughts. He was relieved that he had
been unable to detect any evil intentions on my part, which I interpreted as positive transference. Although the delusional symptoms did
not change to any great extent during the first 9 months, his ego functions stabilized sufficiently that he was able to attend school again. The
therapeutic relationship served as his secure base; he came to therapy
sessions regularly and arrived punctually. The delusional symptoms
changed over time to the point where he could discuss "God and the
world," transcendence, and close and distant attachments and relationships at great length and in a more differentiated way. From then on, he
also became more able to look at his relationship to his parents in a differentiated way. However, he could make absolutely no connection between the sphere of his relationship with his parents and his own fantasy world. He oscillated between two worlds: identifying increasingly
once more with the religious world of his mother, from which he criticized his "faithless" father and his interest in rationality and technology; he also identified with his father's technological world, and from
this position he criticized the mother's "superstition." He thus oscillated
between the two parents, identifying with one or the other at various
times.

During this time, his delusional symptoms were abating; toward
the end of the second year of treatment, the patient was increasingly

able to follow his own path. A relationship with a close friend, with whom he had previously spent hours putting together technological devices, gained in importance during this time. He could now withdraw to his room with his friend, thereby creating a boundary between himself and his parents, while at the same time not withdrawing into solitude with his computer. In the therapeutic relationship, he now seemed more like an adolescent who wants to get into deep intellectual discussions in order to "understand the world." He was very critical of me in his arguments, rejecting my ideas about how things work, and increasingly creating boundaries between us. He confronted me with clear direct questions about "God and the world" that he actually wanted to have answered. He challenged me to take a position, to "show my colors," as a way of structuring the relationship with me, and our negotiations over identification and boundaries. It was not possible to use the classical technique of restating the patient's questions back to him; he would have interpreted this as direct avoidance of attachment, rejection, and withdrawal. What was needed was a "goal-corrected" partnership suited to adolescents in which common goals could be discussed and clarified, and in which each partner could set his own boundaries and express his own opinions. This friendly back-and-forth, set against a backdrop of growing attachment, allowed him to deal with his mother and father as though he had used the therapy sessions to test in advance how far he could go with his thoughts and ideas. Over the course of his further development, these ideas became more realistic, while at the same time sharply intellectual and complex; this kind of thinking was a method that he used "as a weapon" for exploration as well as for setting boundaries.

Treatment ended when he decided to pursue professional training of which neither the mother nor the father approved. He fought to have his way even though he was convinced that his decision would "disappoint" both parents. It was important to him that a therapist could follow and share in his decision.

*Concluding Remarks and Follow-Up*

From a therapeutic perspective, treatment had not been brought to a conclusion at the time that O. decided to go his own way and terminate.

It became clear that he also needed to separate from me as a parental figure, and to go his own way. I had misgivings about how stable he was and whether or not his psychotic symptoms would recur. His parents called and told me that he had been able to pursue his chosen goal without any renewal of his psychosis, to their amazement and to my surprise.

At the same time, we need to deal with our reservation about whether this newly won psychic stability might be insufficient to maintain itself under greater stress. On the basis of diagnostic criteria, therapists may frequently consider that a treatment is not successfully ended because this or that issue still could to be worked through. Perhaps it is necessary to allow patients to terminate treatment when they believe themselves to be secure enough to try, even though there is the potential and the danger that their symptoms may recur. If the attachment relationship in therapy is robust, patients can always return to it. If they do, they may get to the point of attempting termination again, and this time succeeding in spite of the stresses involved.

## Depression in Old Age

*Initial Presentation and Symptoms*

I got to know Mrs. P. while she was an inpatient, hospitalized for several weeks for "severe depressive symptoms." The differential diagnosis included incipient dementia. Mrs. P. was known on the unit for sitting virtually immobile in her chair all day long; it was unclear what she took in from her surroundings. She said nothing and seemed not to be interested in anyone. Watching her, one got the feeling that she was in a stupor, inaccessible to outsiders either emotionally or cognitively.

*Patient History*

Until her inpatient admission, Mrs. P. had shared an apartment with her daughter. At the daughter's disclosure that she planned to marry soon, and that it would be best if the mother went to a nursing home, Mrs. P. at first protested, complained, and raged vociferously. The next morning, however, she failed to get out of bed and had not spoken a word since. At first she was thought to have had a stroke, but no pathological findings were found in neurological tests. Because of this, an acute crisis or a severe depressive reaction were assumed; later came the consideration of incipient dementia. Still, such acute symptoms in connection with a triggering event were not consistent with dementia. Mrs. P. had always lived with her daughter, and they formed a smoothly functioning team; Mrs. P. did the housekeeping while her daughter worked all day. She could not conceive that her daughter might get married and that she would have to spend her waning years in a nursing home. A fragmentary patient history was taken from the daughter, because the mother herself still would not say a word about her person or her life. My initial attempts to engage Mrs. P. and talk to her hit a blank wall. The tiny white-haired 75-year-old woman squinted piercingly at me from behind her wire-rimmed glasses. I had a strong feeling that she perceived me, but she didn't react with words, gestures, or facial expressions, and she certainly did not answer my questions. Nevertheless, I was fascinated and affected by this patient, who lived on the unit like a silent statue. I noticed that I looked at her more often, and felt emotionally involved with her. I wondered what lay hidden behind her silence.

*Consideration of Attachment Dynamics*

First of all, it is notable that the illness with its depressive symptoms began when her daughter spoke of an imminent separation. The announcement that she wanted to get married and that her mother would have to go to a nursing home obviously triggered so much fear and terror in the patient that after a short protest, as her daughter had described, she was rendered speechless in the truest sense of the word. The mother's speechlessness, and her depressive withdrawal, meant that the daughter had to look after her mother and was therefore not in a position to get married and build her life as she intended. The daughter was very frightened by her mother's illness, the initial uncertainty about her condition, and the suspicion that a stroke might have occurred. The entanglement between daughter and mother became even more intense as a result. Several months had elapsed in the meantime. Inpatient treatment (including both psychotherapy and medication) for severe acute depression did nothing to help break through her silence. By then, Mrs. P. was showing signs of hospitalism; she was a part of the unit, but not much attention was paid to her. She existed inconspicuously and caused no trouble. Her daughter visited her regularly several times per week. The daughter herself needed psychotherapeutic help as well because of her guilt feelings about her marriage plans and the separation that would result. From an attachment perspective, one would speculate that mother and daughter represented a secure base to each other, but of very limited scope. The boundaries were demarcated in such a way that there was no room for autonomy and exploration. Their living arrangement had so far made this unnecessary. But the entire situation was shaken by the daughter's intention to marry. Even the thought of separation and the potential expansion of her own scope of exploration brought about the mother's severe reactive depression. The consequence was that her attachment to the daughter became more anxious, making actual separation impossible. At first I was not at all clear why, and in what personal context, this attachment relationship had developed into such a close collusion. Therefore I had no clear idea how to work with this patient, particularly as she reacted to my various attempts at interaction with complete silence and immobility.

*Therapy and Course*

Even though Mrs. P. appeared not to react expressively, I nevertheless considered it necessary from the point of view of attachment at least to maintain contact with her and not to view her as a living statue on the unit. I tried to do this first by visual contact and then by talking to her repeatedly, without expecting any form of verbal expression from her in response. I suspected from her eye movements that she heard me, understood, and wanted to be talked to as well. I got the impression that she wanted to catch my eye when we sat together in a circle with other patients.

One day the staff and patients went out on an excursion, and Mrs. P. went along. As we were strolling through the town, I noticed that she seemed to shadow me, even though she kept a certain distance. It was as if there were an invisible bond of long standing between us. As we walked by a music store, I saw a beautiful old instrument in the window. I left the group and went inside, wanting to look at it more closely. The group, the staff members, and I set a time when we would meet at the train station. I played the instrument for a while and noticed that Mrs. P. was sitting behind me listening. The instrument fascinated me, and I was a little irritated that the patient had followed me. I had also lost track of time and was shocked when I looked at my watch. I said, "Oh my God, we missed the train," to which Mrs. P. answered calmly, speaking for the first time, "That doesn't matter. We have a lot to talk about."

I was completely confused but very moved. Mrs. P. had spoken to me. We walked together in silence to the train station and asked about the next train. Then we sat down to wait for it, across from each other at a small table in a café. Without prompting, Mrs. P. began to talk about how she and her husband, who was a musician, had traveled around the world during the war. In the end, after all of the ravages of the war, she had lost him anyway. Only her daughter, her "everything," remained. She continued to love her husband in her daughter. Until now, she had buried her grief at the loss of her beloved husband deep inside her. Her eyes welled with tears as she related her life story, and I now understood that the idea of separating from her daughter meant that she would have to not only grieve that loss but also make up for a 30-year delay in mourning her husband. When I played the instrument, her memories of him had been so vividly awakened that, given the attachment that had already been cautiously established between us, she became ready to break her silence and talk to me about these matters. Until then it had not been possible; the burden she felt in her heart was simply too great, and each word had been too much for her.

This very emotional event strengthened the attachment between us, which enabled us to do grief work. Over time, I realized that the patient's looks reminded me of my grandmother, who had once been an important attachment figure for me. Her condition improved to the point where she was soon able to discuss with her daughter the possibility of going into a home. It was very important for Mrs. P. to find some sort of assisted living and not simply be "shunted aside" in a nursing home. One condition was that she should be permitted to bring her own furniture, antiques that had become very dear to her, to her new home as a symbolic representation of bygone days. Once an appropriate home was found and she went successfully through a trial period there, we planned her discharge from the clinic and she moved to the new place. Mrs. P. carefully selected the pieces of furniture and mementos she would bring with her into this new, if more constricted, home. She continued to come for therapy on an outpatient basis; it focused on grief work, over both the separation from her daughter and the untimely loss of her husband. Mrs. P. was able to look back over her entire life. It was as if she were separating from old attachments and entering a new world. As a result, she was able to make contact with others in her new living situation and enter into new attachments and relationships.

*Concluding Remarks and Follow-Up*

Mrs. P. became a very valued and engaged member of the community, taking part in a number of activities there. We corresponded for many years, and she described her new life to me in long letters. She joyfully reported her grandchildren's development and was full of pride about how they were thriving and all the things they could do. When she died many years later, and I received an obituary from the daughter, I was very saddened even though her passing, preceded by a brief illness, did not come as a complete surprise.

~

## SUMMARY

I will now summarize several basic ideas that have been developed in these case presentations.

Establishing a secure attachment relationship ("secure base") with the patient was an important therapeutic task in every case. This process is a prerequisite for enabling the patient to change pathological childhood representations of self and attachment figures through work in the transference.

During their hospitalizations, the patients almost certainly experienced staff members, other patients, or the clinic itself as such a "secure base." Special difficulties were associated with establishing and structuring a secure attachment relationship with patients who demonstrated an insecure–avoidant, or dismissing, attachment strategy. My attempts to establish an attachment relationship were particularly unsuccessful with patients of this kind when there was no pressure because the patient did not feel he was suffering, or when parents with avoidant attachment strategies did not want to commit to therapy for their ill child and I was unable to convince them of the need.

An understanding of the various attachment patterns made it easier for me to understand the patients' attachment disorders and enabled me to tailor my technique accordingly. However, these cases also make it clear that clinical variations in attachment disorders at the level of behavior and symptom may deviate considerably from the patterns of insecure attachment identified through research with nonclinical groups.

After therapy, the patients were able to structure their relationships in ways that were more or less symptom-free, and that allowed them greater flexibility in attachment and autonomy as well as in exploring the external and the intrapsychic worlds. I consider this as a sign that their inner working models of relating had changed in the direction of a secure attachment pattern, and that a clearer structure and hierarchy among the working models had been achieved. One indicator of this was patients' ability to replace maladaptive with adaptive attachment behavior. The secure base offered by therapeutic attachment allowed them to work through relationship conflicts and to express and integrate loving and hostile affects in the transference with less anxiety.

Other attachment figures in the patients' environment, such as spouses or parents, may be regarded as either protective or risk factors. Over the course of therapy these relationships must be explored by the patient. Especially in cases of insecure–ambivalent and entangled attachment relationships, such as may occur between spouses or between parents and child, illness may be triggered in a previously healthy person if one partner develops more autonomy over the course of therapy and becomes increasingly able to set boundaries in the relationship.

A certain vulnerability with regard to issues of attachment, separation, and loss remains for patients, despite their new attachment experiences in therapy. Several of the follow-up histories showed that patients who had terminated therapy sought me out again on their own when experiencing a recurrence of symptoms or stress. I also experienced patients after therapy as being more self-reflective and knowledgeable in analyzing a particular attachment dynamic in the context of dealing with a new set of problems.

In several shorter, more focused therapy situations, I did not attempt to terminate the relationship at the end of treatment, so that the patients would feel that they could fall back on me as a secure base if at a later date they encountered anxiety-provoking or threatening situations. Some of them actually did so. Sometimes, however, I made a great effort toward the end of therapy to work toward a permanent termination in order to promote the development of the patient's own autonomy and relatedness to others. Notwithstanding, several patients called me again, something that I initially thought to stem from an inadequately worked-through separation from me. Today (in retrospect and with greater knowledge of attachment theory), I interpret this to mean that attachment within the therapeutic relationship also remains a lifelong issue. In those cases in which I actually succeeded in establishing a secure base with the patient in the relationship, I no longer see it as a sign of "failed therapy" or "inadequate working through" when patients in trouble turn to me again later on.

To the extent that we commit to treatment and place ourselves at the patient's disposal as a secure base, each step that the patient makes toward a new perspective on life, and each farewell at the end of therapy, requires that we also partake in separation and grief work. This process is all the more intense and painful when it resonates with aspects of our own attachment experiences. We must be conscious of our own attachment strategies and countertransference processes so that we do not hold back the development of a patient's autonomy out of our own attachment needs. This danger is particularly great when therapists live alone or (occasionally because of professional involvements) neglect their own personal attachment relationships. In my experience, good attachment-oriented therapy is possible only if therapists are part of a network of relationships that represent a secure base in their own lives and for their own emotional attachments. This will help them to let go of their patients, but it will not spare them the necessity of their own grief work when their patients leave them.

# Section V

~

# Prospects for Further Application

The case studies show that attachment processes represent a challenge that may begin before birth—perhaps even before conception—and endure into old age. The development of attachment is by no means limited to the first year of life. Attachment and exploration, as well as the development of autonomy that is bound up with them, are the poles of a developmental dynamic that is active throughout life.

We must alert parents, teachers, and social workers to the importance of attachment as a fundamental motive force in life, so that this understanding may be put to use in education and in psychotherapy. On reaching developmental milestones—as when an infant learns to walk, or to exert its own will, or as when an adolescent demands greater autonomy—attachment needs may also strongly come to the fore. Completely normal growth crises may result from the tensions inherent in such phases.

Given this theoretical background, it should be possible to do preventive work with expectant parents. Anna Buchheim and I started a training program for parents in Ulm based on this idea. We organized five evening groups, in which we gave first-time expectant parents in the third trimester of pregnancy information from infant research. These sessions dealt particularly with issues of attachment and separation, which we explained with examples. We also integrated a self-assessment component, so that parents could examine their own concepts of and experiences with attachment and separation. After delivery, we saw the mother and father individually with the infant. We made a video recording of the parents diapering and playing with their infant. Then we analyzed the tape together with the parents. The goal of this training was to improve the parents' perception and interpretation of their child's signals, in order to sensitize them to their own behavior.

Our experience indicates that such training does not meet the needs of parents who have attachment disorders of their own. Nevertheless, it did prepare young parents to seek therapeutic help when they encountered difficulties in this sphere. Our program was a first attempt to ensure that early childhood development, and the necessary education of parents about it, not be left to chance. Parents often feel abandoned and overburdened because they lack experience. Sometimes they despair, as they see their attempts to establish an attachment relationship with their child run into a dead end. This may make them fearful of another pregnancy. Sometimes they hope that they have learned from their mistakes, and so look forward to a second pregnancy. However, because their own attachment dynamics will not have changed greatly, variations of the same attachment and relational drama will be played out with the next child as well.

Since having secondary attachment figures may serve as a protective factor for a child, it may be helpful to encourage parents from the beginning to deepen their relationships with such secondary figures for the child as friends, aunts, grandparents, and frequent baby-sitters. It is important to select these people carefully, and to determine how far they are able to commit to an attachment to a child. Only if this is done can such secondary attachment figures be positive forces in the development of secure attachment (cf. also Brisch et al., 1997).

Information and training in the principles of attachment theory, particularly in therapeutic and educational settings, may make it possible for professionals who work in those settings to open up entirely new ways of thinking. As a result, they may be better able to understand children's transition to preschool or elementary school, and to assess their learning processes and peer interactions.

The task of getting used to new surroundings in childhood (family moves, for instance, or starting school or daycare) and even during adulthood (job changes, entering an old age home) could be structured in accordance with attachment theory. This might mean, for example, that the mother would stay with the child and help care for him when he is first starting daycare until he has gotten used to the new situation. Separation periods could then be lengthened as the child begins to form an attachment to the daycare provider on which he can rely in his own mother's absence. This process of acclimatization and the establishment of new attachment relationships require time, particularly in infancy and early childhood, and cannot be rushed (Laewen, Andres, & Hédevári, 1990).

Adolescence is another important threshold during which attachment behaviors are activated in conjunction with demands for autonomy. It is particularly important to educate parents about adolescence and to provide for them a place in which they can talk about their own needs for attachment and the anxiety they feel about their youngster's growing independence. Then any attachment difficulties that may have occurred earlier will be less likely to be reenacted. Thus, an adolescent crisis can present a chance to revise, or to further develop, inner working models.

The final case study shows that separation processes can be worked through even in old age if one is able to focus on relevant attachment principles. Even older people can be uprooted and moved if sufficient time and space are allotted for them to develop new attachments and to work through the processes of separation and grief. However, this requires that everyone involved understand the significance of attachment and separation—especially adult children who often press for separation and transfer of aging parents to nursing homes, but also the staff employed in such homes.

There has been increasing concern about aggressive behavior and violence in preschools and schools. Even though the findings of studies on the growing incidence of violence are not unequivocal, there is a great deal of evidence that the forms taken by aggressive arguments and behaviors among schoolchildren have changed considerably, such that violent acts continue even after a schoolmate lies bloodied on the ground. The ability to empathize with others appears either to have been completely lost, or may possibly never have existed.

Attachment research demonstrates that preschool children who received avoidant attachment classifications with their mothers during the Strange Situation in infancy tend to produce aggressive resolutions when asked to comment on drawings depicting ambiguous interactive situations. Children who were classified as securely attached, in contrast, produce prosocial resolutions. This finding has led to discussions of whether a secure attachment at age 1 is a protective factor, in terms of fostering subsequent prosocial behavior with peers. Securely attached children may perhaps be able to feel their way more empathically and sensitively into another person's world and find constructive resolutions to conflicts precisely because they are able to empathize (Suess et al., 1992).

Researchers on aggression, particularly Henry Parens (1993b), proceed from the assumption that there is such a thing as prosocial aggression or assertiveness—the kind that takes place during exploration or in seeking connection with others—that may be differentiated from destructive aggression. The former accords with Lichtenberg's (1989) exploratory motivation and Bowlby's (1969) attachment–exploration balance. According to Parens, the destructive type of aggression arises from the experience of extreme frustration. This may occur when children have needs for age-appropriate care that are not adequately met when they are prevented from engaging in healthy exploration, or when attachment disorders prevent them from finding appropriate resolutions (cf. the case examples in Section IV for more). It is possible to understand the rage, disappointment, and finally aggression that a 1-year-old avoidantly attached child must suppress in order not to express his natural need for attachment to his mother. One can further imagine that these feelings, associated as they are with considerable physiological tension (Spangler & Schieche, 1995), may be diverted to other relationships. In such circumstances, small frustrations may serve as an igniting "spark." This model might also explain the tendency to act out with considerable aggression for seemingly trivial reasons.

However, it is also possible that children with extreme attachment disorders have lost the ability to feel their way sensitively and empathically into the emotional world of others as a result of their experience of their parents' insensitive behavior. A child from such a background might understandably continue to beat a helpless schoolmate who poses no further threat.

For reasons like these, early training of preschoolers and elementary school students in sensitivity and empathy might represent a corrective emotional experience. It would facilitate understanding of the defensively excluded aggressive feelings they develop in their attachment to their parents and other attachment figures, and help them acquire a capacity for empathy and for establishing new connections. This could possibly have a corrective effect.

With this as a backdrop, Parens (1993a, 1993c; Parens & Kramer, 1993) began to offer a very well designed program of sensitivity and empathy training in preschools. The preschoolers were visited by unfamiliar mothers and their infants. With appropriate supervision, they learned to observe the mother–child interaction, to describe it, and in this way to feel themselves into the infant's world.

Children who had successfully completed such a program reacted to each other with considerably greater sensitivity and prosocial behavior than children in a control group. Parens developed similar programs for elementary schools and high schools, with very elaborate lesson plans, including age-appropriate learning goals and methods appropriate to achieve them. In each case, the goal was for the children to feel their way into the other person and to develop conflict resolution strategies.

If larger-scale preventive programs drawing on the insights of attachment theory could be introduced in preschools, we might be able to counteract aggression and violence in schools. In addition, such work might offer long-term emotional and cognitive corrective experiences to at-risk children from difficult family circumstances.

It would be highly desirable, from a prevention perspective, if all who deal with the early development of infants and children—parents expecting a first child, physicians, teachers, psychologists, social workers, midwives, pediatric nurses, child psychotherapists—were familiar with the basic principles of attachment theory. The use of these principles could potentially prevent attachment disorders from occurring in the first place. In other cases, appropriate action could be taken at an early stage; sensitive interaction with a secondary attachment figure, for example, might lead to a secure attachment with that figure and greater trust in others. This is the goal of a variety of studies of attachment-oriented intervention (Bakermans-Kranenburg et al., 1998).

~

## FAMILY THERAPY

The systems approach to family therapy deals primarily with the invisible bonds and loyalties among family members. Concepts of attachment and autonomy have played a considerable theoretical and interpretive role in its practice.

Early in his career, Bowlby (1949) said that both parental and family relationships must be taken into consideration when children are in psychotherapy, and he invited parents into therapy with their children. This idea has been developed further such that all interactions within the family were interpreted from the perspective of attachment theory (Sroufe & Fleeson, 1988).

Byng-Hall (1991; Byng-Hall & Stevenson-Hinde, 1991) examined the various attachment relationships within the family from the perspective of a so-called family script that encompasses in principle the various working models of family members in dyads and their respective interplays. The family script notion deals with the way roles are distributed for getting and giving help and support within the family, and with how these processes are represented, and thus affect expectations about attachment behavior in the family. Particular diagnostic issues of concern are whether individual family members are excluded from the family attachment system and whether individuals achieve their attachment security at the cost of others.

The concept of "parentification," or, to use Bowlby's (1980) phrase, "inverting the parent–child relationship," is particularly important in this regard. It refers to a parent's use of a child as his or her own "secure base," so that the child must suppress his own needs for caregiving by the parent. Relatedly, children can take on the function of distance and closeness "regulators" in relationships. Particularly when the parents' marriage is difficult, they may do this by developing symptoms that force the parents to maintain their attachment relationship to each other in order to care for the sick child. It is easy to understand why parents in this situation might not permit the child's desire for autonomy, which implies exploration outside of the family.

When a family in crisis comes to the first family therapy session for help, the attachment system of each individual family member is activated, revealing the interplay of attachment patterns within the family. It is not easy for the family therapist to gain the trust of each individual family member so that therapy may proceed. If the therapist is successful in doing so, however, the chances improve that a family will commit to a process of emotional change in the therapeutic setting, and the therapist himself becomes a part of the extended family attachment system.

In order to strengthen this incipient attachment process between therapist and family members, Byng-Hall (1991) suggests that sufficient time must be allotted to the first session (2 hours or more), and that the family should be seen weekly during the initial phase of treatment. Once therapeutic bonds have been established, the interval between appointments may be increased.

One of the fundamental tasks of therapy is to assist the family in establishing for itself a script that reflects the qualities of a "goal-corrected system." By this I mean that each family member must be able to experience the fulfillment of attachment needs for closeness, security, protection from danger, and safety within the family system while at the same time being allowed autonomy to engage in exploration within, and especially outside, the family.

Over the past several years, there has been extensive basic research into the significance of attachments within the family system as a whole (Stevenson-Hinde, 1990). The results are expected to shape future research projects, such as those relating to the prevention of domestic violence (Byng-Hall & Stevenson-Hinde, 1991).

~

## GROUP PSYCHOTHERAPY

According to Lichtenberg (1989), there is a specific motivational system for attachment to a group. This idea is not new; however, it is not receiving attention in proportion to its importance. Presently, group psychotherapy makes up a rather small percentage of the number of patients in outpatient psychotherapy in Germany. This is undoubtedly due to legal issues relating to insurance and billing, and is all the more regrettable because human attachment processes do not operate solely in dyads. Attachment develops, also, to groups—initially to the family, then to a larger extended family, and finally to neighborhoods and even to country. Many findings in social research allow us to conclude that human beings are basically social creatures. For this reason, group psychotherapy based on attachment theory should be promoted in combination with individual therapy, or as a continuation of individual therapy. Such a procedure is often integrated into inpatient therapeutic settings, but unfortunately it has been little used in outpatient treatment. In group psychotherapy it is often possible to observe how patients who are new to the group are accepted by the other group members only after a warm-up period, and how they must feel safe in the group before it can serve them as an attachment "matrix" from which they can derive security. Only then will the patient be able to open himself emotionally to the group members and to explore his (and their) anxiety-provoking issues.

The classical analytical setting of group psychotherapy, where there is often silence and the therapist also may be silent or reticent, is unlikely to create a situation in which new participants may establish a secure group attachment, in the sense of "This is my group, and I belong here" (Schain, 1989).

~

## EDUCATION

If one considers, as attachment theory proposes, that attachment and exploration are interdependent, then one comes to appreciate the importance of attachment theory for education. Under optimal circumstances, the establishment of a secure relationship with a teacher can compensate for deficits with primary attachment figures and at the same time increase curiosity and the willingness to learn. Knowledge of the tenets of attachment theory can help teachers to better understand the interactional processes between themselves and individual students as well as within the class as a whole.

Although the teacher can be seen as an attachment figure during elementary school years, because the students remain in the same class with him or her, the importance of any individual teacher decreases as the students advance to middle school and high school, because there are different teachers for each of the various subjects. Viewed this way, it is understandable that students who switch into a new school that they find intimidating may become emotionally disturbed and do poorly in class, because they cannot find the security they need for optimal learning.

A student who feels safe in a group and with the teacher may be able to enter more successfully into the learning process. Unfortunately, however, our present school system and our society as a whole are organized to avoid attachment. The student who pays little attention to relationships, enters into a few attachments, and is oriented to performance is probably seen as the ideal and receives the most encouragement. Teachers often have the idea that it "saves trouble" to just "stick to the material" and behave in class in a manner that avoids their students' attachment. This technique will cause few problems with attachment–avoidant students. However, all other students—those who look to the teacher for a secure attachment relationship, and especially children with ambivalent attachments to a parent—will challenge a teacher who behaves like this, demanding both caregiving behavior and emotional relatedness. They won't always do this directly or verbally, but rather indirectly and by creating disturbances (for more, see also the case "Attachment Disorders in School-Age Children, Aggressive Attachment Behavior," pages 149–153).

The same principles apply to psychoeducational work with children and adolescents, as discussed with regard to attachment-oriented psychotherapy. However, psychoeducation must be tailored to the setting according to specific circumstances, and modified as needed.

~

# CRITICAL ISSUES

In principle, attachment theory can be applied to all symptoms, diagnoses, and therapeutic approaches. Because attachment must be seen as a fundamental motivation, and because the development of attachment relationships is a lifelong process, in treating any patient one must at least consider whether there might be a disorder of the attachment system. However, this does not mean that an attachment disorder is present in every mental illness. It is certainly possible that other motivational areas may be disturbed or that they are the main focus of a disorder (Lichtenberg et al., 1992). In this context, I mention disorders of group attachment or basic physiological needs. There may also be sexual motivational disorders of the sort that Freud assumed to be the primary focus of disorders and conflicts, and which to this day are seen as central to psychoanalysis. There may also be disturbances specifically related to destructive aggression.

In this volume I have tried to show how the principles of attachment theory may be put into practice in psychotherapeutic work. The cases are meant to serve as illustrations of technique based on attachment theory. However, attachment theory and its therapeutic applications should not be seen as a panacea, nor can attachment theory serve to explain the origins of all symptoms. Attachment should, however, be seen as a fundamental human motivation that is well documented in the research literature and that is reflected in all therapeutic processes. As such, it requires attention when treating attachment disturbances. Of course, other therapies may involve completely different focuses, and other symptoms may be explained using very different therapeutic models. Attachment-oriented therapy should therefore not be seen as a substitute for other approaches to therapy. Rather, it is a complement that in some cases is best able to explain patient behavior, and therefore to suggest new therapeutic techniques.

It is still an open question whether the preventive and other potential extensions of attachment theory outlined here can be effectively incorporated into an attachment-oriented therapy. The point is not to found a new therapeutic school but rather to follow Bowlby by integrating attachment theory into preventive and therapeutic practice, such that attachment comes to be seen as a self-evident and fundamental interpersonal motivation in all relationships, both therapeutic and otherwise.

There are few available standard criteria for selecting teachers and therapists, or for testing suitability for a chosen profession. The ability or fundamental potential for entering into secure attachment relationships might represent such a selection criterion, and it is one that has so far not been sufficiently appreciated. For example, appropriate research might demonstrate whether a candidate's attachment strategy becomes secure–autonomous over the course of therapeutic training—that is, from the beginning to the end of the training analysis. If not, perhaps we should doubt whether a therapist with an avoidant or markedly ambivalent attachment strategy would be capable—at least if intending to work with an attachment-oriented approach—of serving patients as a secure attachment base of the sort needed for healing to occur.

In my opinion, an intuitive understanding of various attachment patterns already plays a role among the physicians who refer patients to therapists. Certain patients are therefore referred to particular therapists, even though the referring physician may not be able to cite objective reasons for his referral (Enke, 1996).

One specific question should be whether it is actually possible to transform a patient's strategy, as measured before therapy, into a more secure one by using a therapeutic approach based on attachment. Initial empirical studies on this issue indicate that an individual's state of mind with respect to attachment may in fact be changed by psychotherapy (Fonagy, Steele, et al., 1995).

It will be the task of clinically oriented attachment research, such as is now being conducted at several clinics and universities, to test the changes described in the case studies in this book for broader clinical significance.

~

# Afterword

## Inge Bretherton

It was at a plenary address at the 1999 Lindauer Therapy Weeks, an annual convention attended by over 3,000 German mental health professionals, that I first heard Karl Heinz Brisch discuss his ideas about the translation of attachment theory into clinical practice. Relying on previous speakers to introduce the theoretical underpinnings, he devoted most of his hour-long talk to the presentation of a number of the case histories that form the major part of this volume. The German version of his book had just come out, and as soon as the talk ended, members of the audience rushed to the conference bookstore and snapped up all of the 300 hot-off-the press copies that the publisher had made available. After reading a copy of the book overnight, it occurred to me that an English translation might be well received by the many English-speaking therapists and analysts who had begun to use attachment theory in their clinical work. I decided to broach the idea of translation with the author and Dr. Lotte Köhler, a German psychoanalyst who had provided support for the book's publication. I found that other participants at the conference had already made similar suggestions. With the cooperation of The Guilford Press, additional funding by InterNationes, a German government foundation, and thoughtful translation by Kenneth Kronenberg, this venture has now become a reality.

For me, the strength of this book lies in the great variety of clinical issues to which an attachment perspective was applied. Brisch describes families unsuccessfully trying to conceive and mothers with severe postpartum depression, young children who refuse to go to preschool, traumatized foster children, psychotic adolescents, adults with marital and work problems, and finally, a touching account of attachment-related conflict between an aged mother and her adult daughter. The presenting problems were psychological, with psychotic manifestations in some cases, and behavioral or psychosomatic in others. In many instances, prior treatment with psychotropic drugs or behavioral therapy had been unsuccessful. The location of treatment also varied, including in-patient care in psychiatric clinics and consultation in the office as well as with staff in residential facilities. The treatment technique ranged from play therapy with children to various forms of "talking" treatment in short- or long-term psychotherapy.

In departing from a more traditional psychodynamic approach, Brisch took his cue from Bowlby's (1988) proposition that it is the therapist's role "to provide the patient with a secure base from which he can explore the various unhappy and painful aspects of his life, past and present" (p. 138). This requires that the therapist attempt to understand the world from the patient's point of view, so that current fantasies ("misconstructions," as Bowlby preferred to call them) and behaviors can be interpreted and given meaning in terms of the patient's attachment history. Following Bowlby's recommendations, Brisch handled the intake and treatment of patients with great flexibility, using his counter-transference reactions as information about what might be troubling the patient and the patient's family. The timing and duration of sessions was tailored to patients' ability to become engaged. Basing his initial diagnoses in part on Main and Goldwyn's (1984/1998) AAI classifications, he uses this information to help the patient toward more constructive relationships and worldviews. Thus, patients whose dismissing approach made it difficult for them to face their underlying emotional conflicts were offered more time between sessions or shorter sessions until they could tolerate more intense exploration of their attachment-related problems, both current and—in the case of adults—intergenerational.

Others who were highly anxious were at first seen very frequently and encouraged to call in when they felt that they could not cope with their anxiety. In the conduct of treatment, Brisch accepted the setting patients found most tolerable, whether it was to sit face to face, lie on the couch with the therapist sitting next to them, or as in classical analysis, with the therapist out of view. The necessity of gaining the trust and cooperation of other family members was also considered, even when these were not actively involved. Brisch's approach to termination was flexible, with offers to call back in crisis situations in many cases. Finally, Brisch had the courage to present cases that, for a variety of reasons, could not be brought to a successful conclusion, but that nevertheless offered interesting insights for future practice. Whereas many therapists may not be able to offer their patients similar choices in their particular work setting, Brisch's work invites creativity not dogmatism in the application of attachment theory.

In addition to illustrating flexible attachment-guided therapy, Brisch's book raises many theoretical issues. Neither Brisch, nor others interested in applications of attachment theory to therapy, have in mind to establish a new attachment therapy school (e.g., Slade, 1999; West & Keller, 1994). The case histories presented in this book nevertheless highlight the need for additional terminology, or, where extant psychodynamic terminology is used, careful consideration of its meaning from within an attachment perspective (for a detailed discussion, see Fonagy, 1999).

Let me illustrate this with an example from the discussion of adolescence. The optimal situation in parent–adolescent relationships, according to attachment theory, is an in-tandem development of attachment and autonomy, such that the adolescent experiences supportive, but not constrictive, caregiving by the parent as greater self-reliance is achieved. When such a pattern is developed, adolescent "boundary setting" is not necessary to achieve individuation. In line with this theoretical position, research has shown that, when asked to discuss topics on which they disagree, secure parents and adolescents listen to and respect each other's views (e.g., Kobak, Cole, Ferenz-Gillies, Fleming, & Gamble, 1993). Boundary setting would be necessary only when parental behaviors are overly interfering and controlling (see some of Brisch's case histories). This is in contrast to prior theories (e.g., A. Freud,

1958), according to which youthful rebellion is the normal way to achieve an independent self. It is also in contrast with the separation/individuation construct proposed by Mahler, albeit for young children (Mahler, Pine, & Bergman, 1975), wherein separation refers to psychological independence. In attachment theory, separation refers to physical separation only, and is not the royal road to autonomy and self-reliance. However, there is no terminology in attachment theory to describe the process whereby a parent and adolescent negotiate the latter's increasing responsibility. There is also no terminology for the process whereby the parental role as primary attachment figure is taken over by a mate, but an adult child's attachment to the parent is not discontinued.

Relatedly, we need more clarification on how the role of therapist as secure base differs from that of parent or partner as secure base. Because the focus in the therapeutic alliance is on the patient rather than the relationship, it is less reciprocal than a parent–child relationship, and considerably less reciprocal than an attachment relationship between adult partners. West and Keller (1994, p. 322) have suggested the term "auxiliary secure base" to capture this difference. It is also not obvious in what sense the therapist plays a secure base role after termination. Brisch explored various options for allowing patients to recontact him in times of crisis, by telephone, letter, renewed appointments, or in thought. He describes the woman with agoraphobia who coped with her anxiety by imagining the therapist sitting beside her as she dared to make her first independent outings in her car. Moreover, even when patients chose not to make use of Brisch's offer for later contact, this does not necessarily imply that the therapeutic relationship has ceased to have supportive meaning for them.

Finally, Brisch's case histories raise the question of how to explain the behavioral, emotional, and representational changes that successful therapy can often bring about. Therapists work both on the relationship level (which can, but need not remain, "procedural") and on the insight level. At the insight level, conscious explorations of attachment and autonomy issues are most likely to lead to conscious changes in the patients' internal working models of self, other, and world, when new procedural models of relationship are constructed at the same time. But how do new working models emerge? A therapist who serves as an effective secure base may make it possible for a patient to consider, albeit cautiously, possible alternative working models of self with current and past attachment figures. Such models of self and relationships with specific and general others may initially be adopted only provisionally, and be tested out a while before relinquishing the old working models as no longer valid. In this sense, internal *working* models are those representations of self, other, and world that are consciously and unconsciously used to guide current interactions with others. The courage to construct new *working* models on the basis of insights gained during therapeutic encounters hence also requires the relinquishment of old *working* models, which are now seen as no longer adequate, even though they may be remembered. These are processes into which only detailed case histories may give us some insight.

## REFERENCES

Bowlby, J. (1988). *A secure base: Parent–child attachment and healthy development.* New York: Basic Books.

Fonagy, P. (1999). Psychoanalytic theory from the viewpoint of attachment theory and research. In J. Cassidy & P. R. Shaver (Eds.), *Handbook of attachment: Theory, research, and clinical applications* (pp. 575–594). New York: Guilford Press.

Freud, A. (1958). Adolescence. *Psychoanalytic Study of the Child, 13,* 255–278.

Mahler, M., Pine, F., & Bergman, A. (1975). *The psychological birth of the human infant.* New York: Basic Books.

Main, M., & Goldwyn, R. (1984/1998). *Adult attachment scoring system and classification system.* Unpublished manuscript, University of California at Berkeley.

Kobak, R. R., Cole, H. E., Ferenz-Gillies, R., Fleming, W. S., & Gamble, W. (1993). Attachment and emotion regulation during mother–teen problem solving: A control theory analysis. *Child Development, 64,* 231–245.

Slade, A. (1999). Attachment theory and research: Implications for the theory and practice of individual therapy with adults. In J. Cassidy & P. R. Shaver (Eds.), *Handbook of attachment: Theory, research, and clinical applications* (pp. 575–594). New York: Guilford Press.

West, M., & Keller, A. (1994). Psychotherapy strategies for insecure attachment in personality disorders. In M. B. Sperling & W. H. Berman (Eds.), *Attachment in adults: Clinical and developmental perspectives* (pp. 313–330). New York: Guilford Press.

# *Appendix*

∽

### BRIEF PRÉCIS OF THE
### ADULT ATTACHMENT INTERVIEW PROTOCOL
### EXCERPTED FROM GEORGE, KAPLAN, AND MAIN (1996)

1.  To begin with, could you just help me to get a little bit oriented to your family—for example, who was in your immediate family, and where you lived?
2.  Now I'd like you to try to describe your relationship with your parents as a young child, starting as far back as you can remember.
3–4. Could you give me five adjectives or phrases to describe your relationship with your mother/father during childhood? I'll write them down, and when we have all five I'll ask you to tell me what memories or experiences led you to choose each one.
5.  To which parent did you feel closer, and why?
6.  When you were upset as a child, what did you do, and what would happen? Could you give me some specific incidents when you were upset emotionally? Physically hurt? Ill?
7.  Could you describe your first separation from your parents?
8.  Did you ever feel rejected as a child? What did you do, and do you think your parents realized they were rejecting you?

---

*Important note.* The AAI **cannot** be conducted on the basis of this brief, modified précis of the protocol, which omits several questions as well as the critical follow-up probes. The full protocol, together with extensive directions for administration, can be obtained by writing to Professor Mary Main, Department of Psychology, University of California at Berkeley, Berkeley, CA 94720. Adapted from George, Kaplan, and Main (1996). Copyright 1996 by the authors. Adapted by permission.

9.  Were your parents ever threatening toward you—for discipline, or jokingly?

10. How do you think your overall early experiences have affected your adult personality? Are there any aspects you consider a setback to your development?

11. Why do you think your parents behaved as they did during your childhood?

12. Were there other adults who were close to you—like parents—as a child?

13. Did you experience the loss of a parent or other close loved one as a child, or in adulthood?

14. Were there many changes in your relationship with parents between childhood and adulthood?

15. What is your relationship with your parents like for you currently?

# Notes

## FOREWORD

1.  It is only recently that two volumes of *Psychoanalytic Inquiry* (Vol. 19, Nos. 4 & 5, 1999) were dedicated to "Attachment Research and Psychoanalysis"; several seminal papers on the same topic were published in the *Journal of the American Psychoanalytic Association* (Vol. 48, No. 4, 2000).
2.  For further details see Stern et al. (1998).

## PREFACE

1.  The video laboratory was provided by support from the German Research Council and the "Sanitätsrat Dr. Emil Alexander Huebner und Gemahlin Stiftung im Stiftungsverband für Deutsche Wissenschaft Essen."

## INTRODUCTION

1.  For a comprehensive overview, the reader is referred to other publications (Goldberg, Muir, & Kerr, 1995; Parkes, Stevenson-Hinde, & Marris, 1991; Spangler & Zimmermann, 1995).
2.  In the interests of simplicity I will henceforth use the masculine form when making general comments and statements. It is to be understood that all statements also apply to female therapists and female patients, etc., in whatever context.

## SECTION I. Attachment Theory and Its Basic Concepts

1.  In the German-speaking countries, Gerd and Renate Biermann have been espe-
    cially indefatigable advocates for changes in visiting hours and for the right of
    parents to be present to care for their children in children's clinics.

2.  For a more detailed description of attachment theory, especially with psycho-
    metric data regarding the methodology of attachment theory as well as the re-
    sults of statistical analyses from various studies, see Buchheim, Brisch, and
    Kächele (1998); Schmidt and Strauß (1996); Spangler and Zimmermann
    (1995); Strauß and Schmidt (1997).

3.  Hereafter, I will also write of an "attachment relationship"; by this I mean the
    specific part of the attachment system contained within the relationship. How-
    ever, according to Emde (1989) the relationship between the parents and their
    child is also determined by a variety of other aspects, such as the communica-
    tion and regulation of affect, the regulation of physiological needs, learning,
    play, and self-control.

4.  The importance for the development of attachment of early interactions be-
    tween mother and infant is reminiscent of the construction proposed by Stern
    (1989). Stern proceeds from the repetitive interactive behavior patterns be-
    tween mother and child, which are internalized and representationally stored
    as general patterns.

5.  According to Stern (1986), the attachment working model consists of many
    different generalized representations of interactions. These constitute the "ba-
    sic building blocks of the working model." Thus, according to Stern, the work-
    ing model is a superordinate structure. New interactional experiences are ab-
    sorbed into the working model; old ones may be extinguished. Using this
    conception, one may imagine change as a reorganization of the working model
    over time.

6.  Proceeding from the perspective of infant research, Lichtenberg (1989) embed-
    ded attachment and exploration into the more comprehensive context of moti-
    vation systems. He mentions the system that regulates physiological require-
    ments (he is thinking particularly of hunger, thirst, and heat regulation, and
    similar bodily needs) as well as the attachment and exploration systems. He
    later expands this into the "self-assertion" system, i.e., the ability of the child
    to experience himself as a competent being, one who can experience himself as
    a motivating or initiating force, as well as into an "aversion" system, i.e., one
    governing the ability to react defensively to threatening and dangerous stimuli,
    and finally into a system governing the satisfaction of sensual and sexual needs.

7.  Studies conducted by Papoušek (1977) have shown that infants are able very
    early on to recognize the connection between external stimuli, their actions,
    and the triggering of reactions. They are capable of actively reproducing these
    reactions, with a notable feeling of efficacy that is accompanied by joyful ex-
    citement.

8. If an infant can already walk at the age of 1 year, but is placed in a 10-square-foot playpen for many hours each day, his need for exploration is not satisfied. On the other hand, if an infant of that age could explore the entire house from cellar to attic, it would be absolutely necessary to set limits. The amount of room for exploration appropriate to the age as well as appropriate limits must be set according to the developmental age of the particular infant, without becoming too loose or too constricting.

9. In my opinion, a precondition for this is that the mother be able to endure her own separation anxiety, which results from the loss of her close relationship to her infant, during this exploration, and not project her own fears onto the infant. On the other hand, she must perceive her infant's anxieties as he moves away, contain them intrapsychically, and "hold" or endure them.

10. This "goal-corrected partnership" develops during childhood and is structured in accordance with the child's needs at a particular age. In a study involving adolescents, Becker-Stoll (1997) studied how these "goal-corrected partnerships" were structured in arguments over vacation planning between the adolescent and the attachment figure.

11. One mother may awaken at the slightest sound from her child; other mothers report that they sleep so soundly that their children may already be standing in their beds screaming in panic before she wakes up and is able to react. However, the level of sensitivity is not only determined by the inner well-being of the mother but also by secondary social conditions. Thus, a mother who is supported by her partner will be better able to concentrate on the needs of her child than a mother who, because she comes home from work dead tired, is hardly able to summon the strength to react to her child's loud crying in an appropriate way.

12. During field studies in Papua New Guinea, mothers were observed to carry their infants on their bodies for most of the day in accordance with tradition. Surprisingly, the researchers never saw infants soiling their mothers. An explanation might be that a sensitive mother perceives her infant's increasing restlessness before a bowel movement (Wulf Schiefenhövel, personal communication). Similar observations were made in East Africa in a study carried out by DeVries and DeVries (1977).

13. The organization of the Institute and the realization of this study were made possible by a research grant from the Köhler-Stiftung Darmstadt, Germany.

14. The incoherence of the dialogue in the following example is not the result of incorrect transcription of the audiotape. The example actually is this confused and clearly reproduces the "entanglement" of the dialogue.

15. Because Anna Freud and Dorothy Burlingham had been involved in the psychotherapeutic treatment of children during the war, greater cooperation with Bowlby on this issue might have developed. Unfortunately, this never occurred.

16. Winnicott also studied the causes of "antisocial tendencies." His ideas show parallels to Bowlby's early theory. Winnicott explained the development of an-

tisocial behavior as a consequence of emotional deprivation because "the [child] in stealing was unconsciously looking for the mother from whom he had the right to steal" (1958, p. 292).

17. Infant research has rendered this theoretical concept untenable. To the contrary, we now assume that the infant is intrapsychically primed for interaction, and that he seeks to test out and establish such interaction with his attachment figure very rapidly and dynamically. During Margaret Mahler's lifetime, the differential perceptive and expressive potentials during the first weeks of life were not yet known and were only available to psychotherapists as a result of advances in research into infant development, and its reception generally and by psychoanalysis in particular.

18. Dornes (1997) pointed out the similarity between children's behavior in the rapprochement crisis described by Mahler and the ambivalent attachment pattern in attachment theory. He doubted that the rapprochement crisis phase is a normal developmental phase in individuation.

19. Freud (1920/1955) had already pointed out the potential ability of the child to symbolize his mother in separation situations. In his work on the pleasure principle, Freud interpreted his 1½–year-old nephew's repeated playing with a ball of yarn as an attempt, in play, to represent separation from his mother, which he was then experiencing, as well as to symbolize the reunion that he desired and process his aloneness intrapsychically.

## SECTION II. Attachment Disorders

1. Today, school phobia is viewed as a disturbance resulting from separation anxiety (ICD-10).

2. This form of attachment disorder with exaggerated clinging is listed by Zeanah (Zeanah & Emde, 1994) as a subtype of "inhibited attachment behavior." However, the designation "exaggerated attachment behavior" seems a more appropriate description to me of the clinical pictures seen with this type of attachment disorder.

3. This type of attachment disorder is an addition of mine. It has not been described in the literature to date.

## SECTION III. Attachment Therapy

1. In the German version, I translated the term "therapeutic bond" as "Bindungs-beziehung zwischen Patient und Therapeut" because it comes closest to what Orlinsky described. Other authors use other terms and translations in this context, such as "therapeutic alliance," which is translated into German as

"therapeutische Allianz" or "therapeutisches Bündnis," although these terms describe more the conscious part of the patient–therapist relationship. The concept of "bond," on the other hand, is directly linked to "bonding" and "attachment" and puts the stress on the attachment aspects within the relationship, including its affective parts.

2.  In trauma therapy, an important precondition for processing trauma is that the therapist makes sufficient time before processing to find a "secure place" with the patient. This imaginary place can be inside or outside the patient, and he seeks out this place in his imagination in moments of great anxiety when the trauma is being activated in order to feel emotional protection and security. An imagined "*inner helping companion*," which is reminiscent of an attachment figure who offers protection, security, and relief from anxiety and takes over *the help-ego function*, is similar to the construct of the "secure base" in attachment theory (Reddemann & Sachsse, 1996).

3.  Sensitive explanations that allow the patient to feel deeply understood can also contribute to strengthening the therapeutic bond (Stuhr, 1993).

4.  One could conceptualize these as contradictory "partial working models," borrowing from the *partial objects* of object relations theory.


## SECTION IV. Treatment Cases from Clinical Practice

1.  For reasons of anonymity, we decided to forgo biographical details if these were not considered to be significant for the understanding of the attachment dynamics and the course of treatment. We used initials ("A," "B," "C," etc.) to indicate persons; however, these were not based on their real names.

2.  German high school students receive a certificate after completion of 10th grade or 13th grade. Only completion of 13 grades fulfills the prerequisites for university admission, the 10th grade (intermediate) certificate qualifies a student for further professional training at various technical colleges.

3.  I base this request for concrete examples on the interview style of the AAI.

4.  For a more comprehensive consideration of this problem from the point of view of attachment dynamics, see Wöller (1998).

5.  It is extremely difficult for mothers of children afflicted with neurodermatitis to take their children's needs into account when giving the necessary skin care prescribed by the pediatrician. Such mothers are under great pressure to rub ointment on their children's skin no matter what, because otherwise the skin symptoms often get worse. The result of deterioration in the condition of the skin is visible to all, so that relatives, friends, and even the pediatrician will comment about the lack of skin care. This places mothers in an impossible dilemma: on the one hand, they are supposed to prevent further skin deterioration by using the ointment; on the other hand, they are supposed to be sensi-

tively attuned to their children's needs, which is hardly compatible with the coercion needed to administer these medical treatments.

6. König (1981) described this security function provided by auxiliary ego figures to patients with anxiety disorders as "steering objects."

~

# References

Adam, K. S., Sheldon-Keller, A. E., & West, M. (1996). Attachment organization and history of suicidal behavior in clinical adolescents. *Journal of Consulting and Clinical Psychology, 64*(2), 264–272.

Ainsworth , M. D. S. (1967). *Infancy in Uganda.* Baltimore: Johns Hopkins University Press.

Ainsworth, M. D. S. (1977). Feinfühligkeit versus Unempfindlichkeit gegenüber Signalen des Babys. In K. E. Grossmann (Ed.), *Entwicklung der Lernfähigkeit in der sozialen Umwelt.* München: Kindler, 98–107.

Ainsworth, M. D. S., Bell, S. M., & Stayton, D. J. (1974). Infant–mother attachment and social development: "Socialization" as a product of reciprocal responsiveness to signals. In M. P. M. Richards (Ed.), *The integration of a child into a social world.* New York: Cambridge University Press, 99–135.

Ainsworth, M. D. S. (1985). Patterns of infant–mother attachments: Antecedents and effects on development. *Bulletin of the New York Academy of Medicine, 61,* 771–791.

Ainsworth, M. D. S., Blehar, M. C., Waters, E., & Wall, S. (1978). *Patterns of attachment: A psychological study of the strange situation.* Hillsdale, NJ: Erlbaum.

Ainsworth, M. D. S., & Wittig, B. A. (1969). Attachment and the exploratory behavior of one-years-olds in a strange situation. In B. M. Foss (Ed.), *Determinants of infant behavior.* New York: Basic Books, 113–136.

Alexander, F., & French, T. M. (1946). *Psychoanalytic therapy.* New York: Rolande.

American Psychiatric Association. (1987). Diagnostic and statistical manual of mental disorders (3rd ed., rev.). Washington, DC: Author.

American Psychiatric Association. (1994). Diagnostic and statistical manual of mental disorders (4th ed.). Washington, DC: Author.

Atkinson, L. (1997). Attachment and psychopathology: From laboratory to clinic. In L. Atkinson & K. J. Zucker (Eds.), *Attachment and psychopathology.* New York: Guilford Press, 3–16.

Bakermans-Kranenburg, M., Juffer, E., & van IJzendoorn, M. H. (1998). Interventions with video feedback and attachment discussions: Does type of maternal insecurity make a difference? *Infant Mental Health Journal, 19*, 202–219.

Balint, M. (1937/1965b). Frühe Entwicklungsstadien des Ichs. Primäre Objektliebe. In *Primary love and psychoanalytic technique*. London: Tavistock.

Balint, M. (1959). *Thrills and regressions*. New York: International Universities Press.

Balint, M. (1961/1965). Beitrag zum Symposium über die Theorie der Eltern-Kind-Beziehung. In *Primary love and psychoanalytic technique*. London: Tavistock.

Barglow, P., Jaffe, C. M., & Vaughn, B. (1988). Psychoanalytic reconstruction and empirical data: Reciproce contribution. *Journal of the American Psychoanalytic Association, 37*, 401–436.

Becker-Stoll, E. (1997). *Interaktionsverhalten zwischen Jugendlichen und Müttern im Kontext längsschnittlicher Bindungsentwicklung*. Unpublished dissertation, Regensburg.

Belsky, J., Rosenberger, K., & Crnic, K. (1995). Maternal personality, marital quality, social support and infant temperament: Their significance for infant–mother attachment in human families. In C. Pryce, R. Martin, & D. Skuse (Eds.), *Motherhood in human and nonhuman primates*. Oxford: Clarendon Press, 193–217.

Belsky, J., & Russell, I. (1988). Maternal, infant, and social-contextual determinants of attachment security. In J. Belsky & T. Nezworski (Eds.), *Clinical implications of attachment*. Hillsdale, NJ: Erlbaum, 41–94.

Benoit, D., & Parker, K. H. C. (1994). Stability and transmission of attachment across three generations. *Child Development, 65*, 1444–1456.

Berlin, M. A. (1991). A comparison of attachment in high-risk preterm and full-term infants using home Q-sort and strange situation assessment methods. *Dissertation Abstracts International, 51*(7-B), 3554-B.

Bion, W. (1962). Eine Theorie des Denkens. In E. Bott Spillius (Ed.), *Melanie Klein Heute, Band 1: Beiträge zur Theorie*. München/Wien: Verlag Internationale Psycboanalyse, 110–129.

Blatz, W (1940). *Hostages to peace: Parents and the children of democracy*. New York: Morrow.

Boszormenyi-Nagy, I., & Spark, G. M. (1973). *Invisible loyalties: Reciprocity in intergenerational family therapy*. New York: Harper & Row.

Bowlby, J. (1946). Forty-four juvenile thieves: Their characters and home life. *International Journal of Psycho-Analysis, 19*–52; 107–127.

Bowlby, J. (1949). The study and reduction of group tension in the family. *Human Relations, 2*, 123.

Bowlby, J. (1951). *Maternal care and mental health*. Geneva: World Health Organization Monograph Series No. 2.

Bowlby, J. (1953). *Child care and the growth of love*. London: Penguin.

Bowlby, J. (1958). The nature of the child's tie to his mother. *International Journal of Psycho-Analysis, 39*, 350–373.

Bowlby, J. (1960a). Grief and mourning in infancy and early childhood. *Psychoanalytic Study of the Child, 15*, 9–52.

Bowlby, J. (1960b). Separation anxiety. *International Journal of Psycho-Analysis, 41*, 313–317.

Bowlby, J. (1969). *Attachment and loss. Vol. 1: Attachment.* New York: Basic Books.

Bowlby, J. (1973). *Attachment and loss. Vol. 2: Separation, anxiety and anger.* New York: Basic Books.

Bowlby, J. (1980). *Attachment and loss. Vol. 3: Loss, sadness and depression.* New York: Basic Books.

Bowlby, J. (1988). *A secure base: Clinical implications of attachment theory.* London: Routledge.

Bowlby, J., Robertson, J., & Rosenbluth, D. (1952). A two-year-old goes to hospital. *Psychoanalytic Study of the Child, 7,* 82–94.

Bretherton, I. (1992). The origins of attachment theory: John Bowlby and Mary Ainsworth. *Developmental Psychology, 28,* 759–775.

Bretherton, I. (1995). Attachment theory and developmental psychopathology. In D. Cicchetti & S. Toth (Eds.), *Emotion, cognition, and representation* (Vol. 6). Rochester, NY: University of Rochester Press, 231–260.

Bretherton, I. (1998, July 6–7). *The development of internal working models of attachment.* Paper presented at the Development, Structure, and Functioning of Internal Working Model Symposium, Universität Regensburg.

Bretherton, I., & Munholland, K. A. (1999). Internal working models in attachment relationships: A construct revisited. In J. Cassidy & P. R. Shaver (Eds.), *Handbook of attachment: Theory, research, and clinical applications.* New York: Guilford Press, 89–111.

Bretherton, I., Oppenheim, D., Buchsbaum, H., & Emde, R. N. (1990). *The MacArthur Story Stem Battery.* Unpublished manuscript, Waisman Center, University of Wisconsin–Madison.

Bretherton, I., Ridgeway, D., & Cassidy, J. (1990). Assessing internal working models of the attachment relationship: An attachment story completion task for 3-year-olds. In M. T. Greenberg, D. Cicchetti, & E. M. Cummings (Eds.), *Attachment in the preschool years.* Chicago: University of Chicago Press, 273–310.

Brisch, K. H. (1998a, June 11–13). *Development of infantile anorexia nervosa and its psychotherapeutic treatment.* International Conference: "The treatment of eating disorders: Research meets clinical practice," Stuttgart.

Brisch, K. H. (1998b). Die Bedeutung der Psychodynamik im Rahmen der pränatalen Fehlbildungsdiagnostik. *Speculum, 16*(1), 23–31.

Brisch, K. H. (2000). The use of the telephone in the treatment of attachment disorders. In J. K. Aronson (Ed.), *Use of the telephone in psychotherapy.* Northvale, NJ: Aronson, 375–395.

Brisch, K. H., Bemmerer-Mayer, K., Munz, D., & Kächele, H. (1998). Angst vor fetaler Fehlbildung und ihre Bewältigung. *Internationale Zeitschrift für pränatale und perinatale Psychologie und Medizin, 10*(3), 349–364.

Brisch, K. H., Buchheim, A., & Kächele, H. (1998, June 4–6). *Bindungsprozesse beim Übergang zur Elternschaft: Beeinflussung der Eltern-Kind-Beziehung durch eine pränatale und postnatale Intervention für erstgebärende Eltern.* 12th Kongreß der Deutschen Gesellschaft für Medizinische Psychologie (DGMP), Hamburg.

Brisch, K. H., Buchheim, A., & Kächele, H. (1999). Diagnostik von Bindungsstörungen. *Praxis der Kinderpsychologie und Kinderpsychiatrie.*

Brisch, K. H., Buchheim, A., Köhntop, B., Kunzke, D., Schmücker, G., Kächele, H., & Pohlandt, E. (1996). Präventives psychotherapeutisches Interventionsprogramm für Eltern nach der Geburt eines sehr kleinen Frühgeborenen— Ulmer Modell. *Randomisierte Längsschnittstudie. Monatsschrift für Kinderheilkunde, 144,* 1206–1212.

Brisch, K. H., Gontard, A. v., Pohlandt, E, Kächele, H., Lehmkuhl, G., & Roth, B. (1997). Interventionsprogramme für Eltern von Frühgeborenen. Kritische Übersicht. *Monatsschrift für Kinderheilkunde, 145,* 457–465.

Buchheim, A., Brisch, K. H., & Kächele, H. (1998). Die klinische Bedeutung der Bindungsforschung für die Risikogruppe der Frühgeborenen: ein Überblick zum neuesten Forschungsstand. *Zeitschrift für Kinder- und Jugendpsychiatrie und Psychotherapie, 27*(2).

Buchheim, A., Brisch, K. H., & Kächele, H. (1998). Einführung in die Bindungstheorie und ihre Bedeutung für die Psychotherapie. *Psychotherapie, Psychosomatik, Medizinische Psychologie, 48,* 128–138.

Byng-Hall, J. (1991). The application of attachment theory to understanding and treatment in family therapy. In C. M. Parkes, J. Stevenson-Hinde, & P. Marris (Eds.), *Attachment across the life cycle.* London: Tavistock, 199–215.

Byng-Hall, J., & Stevenson-Hinde, J. (1991). Attachment relationships within a family system. *Infant Mental Health Journal, 12*(3), 187–200.

Carlson, V., Cicchetti, D., Barnett, D., & Braunwald, K. G. (1989). Finding order in disorganization: Lessons from research on maltreated infants' attachments to their caregiver. In D. Cicchetti & V. Carlson (Eds.), *Child maltreatment: Theory and research on the causes and consequences of child abuse and neglect.* Cambridge: Cambridge University Press, 494–528.

Cassidy, J. (1988). The self as related to child–mother attachment at six. *Child Development, 59,* 121–134.

Cassidy, J., & Shaver, P. R. (Eds.). (1999). *Handbook of attachment: Theory, research, and clinical applications.* New York: Guilford Press.

Cicchetti, D., & Toth, S. L. (1995). Child maltreatment and attachment organization: Implications for intervention. In S. Goldberg, R. Muir, & J. Kerr (Eds.), *Attachment theory: Social, developmental, and clinical perspectives.* Hillsdale, NJ: Analytic Press, 279–308.

Cierpka, M. (1996). Handbuch der Familiendiagnostik. Heidelberg: Springer.

Cole-Detke, H., & Kobak, R. (1994). *Attentional processes in eating disorders and depression: An attachment perspective.* Newark: Department of Psychology, University of Delaware.

Crittenden, P. M. (1985). Maltreated infants: Vulnerability and resilience. *Journal of Child Psychology and Psychiatry and Allied Disciplines, 26,* 85–96.

Crittenden, P. M. (1988). Relationships at risk. In J. Belsky & T. Nezworski (Eds.), *Clinical implications of attachment.* Hillsdale, NJ: Erlbaum, 136–176.

Crittenden, P. M. (1995). Attachment and psychopathology. In S. Goldberg, R. Muir, & J. Kerr (Eds.), *Attachment theory: Social, developmental, and clinical perspectives.* Hillsdale, NJ: Analytic Press, 367–406.

Crittenden, P. M. (1997). Patterns of attachment and sexual behavior: Risk of dysfunction versus opportunity for creative integration. In L. Atkinson & K. J. Zucker (Eds.), *Attachment and psychopathology*. New York: Guilford Press, 47–93.

Crockenberg, S. B. (1981). Infant irritability, mother responsiveness, and social support influences on the security of infant–mother attachment. *Child Development, 52,* 857–869.

Crockenberg, B. (1986). Are temperamental differences in babies associated with predictable differences in care giving? In J. V. Lerner & R. M. Lerner (Eds.), *Temperament and social interaction in infants and children: New directions for child development*. San Francisco: Jossey-Bass, 53–72.

Cummings, E. M. (1990). Classification of attachment on a continuum of felt security: Illustrations from the study of children of depressed parents. In M. T. Greenberg, D. Cicchetti, & E. M. Cummings (Eds.), *Attachment in the preschool years*. Chicago: University of Chicago Press, 311–338.

Cummings, E. M., & Cicchetti, D. (1990). Toward a transactional model of relations between attachment and depression. In M. T. Greenberg, D. Cicchetti, & E. M. Cummings (Eds.), *Attachment in the preschool years*. Chicago: University of Chicago Press, 339–374.

Degkwitz, R., Helmchen, H., Kockott, G., & Mombour, W. (Eds.). (1975). *Diagnosenschlüssel und Glossar psychiatrischer Krankheiten. ICD-8* (4th ed.). Berlin/Heidelberg/New York: Springer.

Degkwitz, R., Helmchen, H., Kockott, G., & Mombour, W. (Eds.). (1980). *Diagnosenschlüssel und Glossar psychiatrischer Krankheiten. ICD-9* (5th ed.). Berlin/Heidelberg/New York: Springer.

De Ruiter, C. (1994). Anxious attachment in agoraphobia and obsessive–compulsive disorder: A literature review and treatment implications. In C. Perris, W. A. Arrindell, & M. Eisemann (Eds.), *Parenting and psychopathology* (pp. 281–307). New York: Wiley.

De Ruiter, C., & von IJzendoorn, M. (1992). Agoraphobia and anxious-ambivalent attachment: An integrative review. *Journal of Anxiety Disorders, 6,* 365–381.

deVries, M. W., & deVries, M. R. (1977). Cultural relativity of toilet training readiness: A perspective from East Africa. *Pediatrics, 60,* 170–177.

De Wolff, M., & van IJzendoorn, M. H. (1997). Sensitivity and attachment: A meta-analysis on parental antecedents of infant attachment. *Child Development, 68,* 571–591.

Dornes, M. (1993). *Der kompetente Säugling*. Frankfurt: S. Fischer.

Dornes, M. (1997). *Die frühe Kindheit. Entwicklungspsychologie der ersten Lebensjahre*. Frankfurt: S. Fischer.

Dornes, M. (1998). Bindungstheorie und Psychoanalyse: Konvergenzen und Divergenzen. *Psyche, 52,* 299–348.

Dozier, M., Stovall, K. C., Albus, K. E., & Bates, B. (2001). Attachment for infants in foster care: The role of caregiver state of mind. *Child Development, 72,* 1467–1477.

Easterbrooks, M. A. (1989). Quality of attachment to mother and to father: Effects of perinatal risk status. *Child Development, 60,* 825–830.

Easterbrooks, M. A., & Goldberg, W. A. (1984). Toddler development in the family: Impact of father involvement and parenting characteristics. *Child Development, 55*, 744–752.

Egeland, B., & Erickson, M. F. (1993). *Final Report: An evaluation of STEEP, a program for high-risk mothers* (Grant No. MH41879). Rockville, MD: National Institute of Mental Health, Department of Health and Human Services.

Emde, R. N. (1989). The infants relationship experience: Developmental and affective aspects. In A. J. Sameroff & R. N. Emde (Eds.), *Relationship disturbances in early childhood: A developmental approach.* New York: Basic Books, 33–51.

Emde, R. N., Oppenheim, D., Nir, A., & Warren, S. (1997). Emotion regulation in mother–child narrative co-construction: Associations with children's narratives and adaptation. *Developmental Psychobiology, 33*, 284–294.

Emde, R. N., & Sorce, J. E. (1983). The rewards of infancy: Emotional availability and maternal referencing. In J. D. Call, E. Galenson, & P. I. Tyson (Eds.), *Frontiers of infant psychiatry.* New York: Basic Books, 17–30.

Enke, H. (1996). Die Zukunft der psychotherapeutischen Ausbildung(en)—Notwendiges und Wünschenswertes. In H. Henning (Ed.), *Kurzzeittherapie in Theorie und Praxis.* Lengenich: Pabst Science, 1188–1196.

Erickson, M. F. (2000). *Seeing is believing (a training video and companion manual).* Minneapolis, MN: Irving B. Harris Training Center for Infant and Toddler Development, University of Minnesota.

Esser, G., Dinter-Jörg, M., Herrle, J., Yantorno-Villalba, P., Rose, F., Laucht, M., & Schmidt, M. H. (1996). Bedeutung der Blickvermeidung im Säuglingsalter für den Entwicklungsstand des Kindes mit zwei und viereinhalb Jahren. *Zeitschrift für Entwicklungspsychologie und Pädagogische Psychologie, 28*, 3–19.

Esser, G., Laucht, M., & Schmidt, M. H. (1995). Der Einfluß von Risikofaktoren und der Mutter-Kind-Interaktion im Säuglingsalter auf die seelische Gesundheit des Vorschulkindes. *Kindheit und Entwicklung, 4*, 33–42.

Finke, J. (1994). *Empathie und Interaktion. Methodik und Praxis der Gesprächspsychotheropie.* Stuttgart/New York: Thieme.

Fonagy, P. (1998). An attachment theory approach to treatment of the difficult patient. *Bulletin of the Menninger Clinic, 62*(2), 147–169.

Fonagy, P., Leigh, T., Kennedy, R., Mattoon, G., Steele, H., Target, M., Steele, M., & Higgit, A. (1995). Attachment, borderline states and the representation of emotions and cognition in self and other. In D. Cicchetti & S. Toth (Eds.), *Emotion, cognition, and representation* (Vol. 6). Rochester, NY: University of Rochester Press, 371–374.

Fonagy, P., Leigh, T., Steele, M., Steele, H., Kennedy, R., Mattoon, G., Target, M., & Gerber, A. (1996). The relation of attachment status, psychiatric classification and response of psychotherapy. *Journal of Consulting and Clinical Psychology, 64*, 22–31.

Fonagy, P., Steele, H., & Steele, M. (1991). Maternal representations of attachment during pregnancy predict the organization of infant–mother attachment at one year of age. *Child Development, 62*, 891–905.

Fonagy, P., Steele, M., Steele, H., Leigh, T., Kennedy, R., Mattoon, G., & Target, M. (1995). Attachment, the reflective self, and borderline states: The predictive specificity of the adult attachment interview and pathological emotional development. In S. Goldberg, R. Muir, & J. Kerr (Eds.), *Attachment theory: Social, developmental, and clinical perspectives.* Hillsdale, NJ: Analytic Press, 233–278.

Fonagy, P., Steele, M., Steele, H., Target, M., & Schachter, A. (1996). *Reflective self-functioning manual for application to Adult Attachment Interview.* Unpublished manual, University College, London.

Fonagy, P., Target, M., Steele, M., Steele, H., Leigh, T., Levinson, A., & Kennedy, R. (1997). Morality, disruptive behavior, borderline personality disorder, crime, and their relationship to security of attachment. In L. Atkinson & K. J. Zucker (Eds.), *Attachment and psychopathology.* New York: Guilford Press, 223–274.

Fox, N. A. (1992). Frontal brain asymmetry and vulnerability to stress: Individual differences in infant temperament. In T. M. Field, P. M. McCabe, & N. Schneiderman (Eds.), *Stress and coping in infancy and childhood.* Hillsdale, NJ: Erlbaum, 83–99.

Fox, N. A. (1995). On the way we were: Adult memories about attachment experiences and their role in determining infant–parent relationships: A commentary on van IJzendoorn (1995). *Psychological Bulletin, 117,* 404–410.

Fox, N. A., Kimmerly, N. L., & Schafer, W. D. (1991). Attachment to mother/attachment to father: A meta-analysis. *Child Development, 62,* 210–225.

Fraiberg, S. (1982). Pathological defenses in infancy. *Psychoanalytic Quarterly, 51,* 623–634.

Fraiberg, S., Adelson, E., & Shapiro, V. (1975). Ghosts in the nursery: A psychoanalytic approach to the problems of impaired infant–mother relationship. *Journal of the American Academy of Child and Adolescent Psychiatry, 14*(3), 387–422.

Freud, A. (1960). Discussion of Dr. John Bowlby's paper. *Psychoanalytic Study of the Child, 15,* 53–62.

Freud, A. (1958, 1960/1969). Discussion of John Bowlby's Arbeit über Trennung und Trauer. In *The writings of Anna Freud.* New York: International Universities Press.

Freud, A. (1980a). Anstaltskinder. Berichte aus den Kriegskinderheimen "Hampstead Nurseries" 1943–1945. In *The writings of Anna Freud.* New York: International Universities Press.

Freud, A. (1980b). Kriegskinder. Berichte aus den Kriegskinderheimen "Hampstead Nurseries" 1941–1942. In *The writings of Anna Freud.* New York: International Universities Press.

Freud, A., & Burlingham, D. (1944). *Infants without families.* New York: International Universities Press.

Freud, S. (1905/1953). Three essays on the theory of sexuality. In J. Strachey (Ed. & Trans.), *The standard edition of the complete psychological works of Sigmund Freud* (Vol. 7). London: Hogarth Press, 123–245.

Freud, S. (1916–1917/1953). Introductory lectures on psycho-analysis. In J. Strachey (Ed. & Trans.), *The standard edition of the complete psychological works of Sigmund Freud* (Vols. 15–16). London: Hogarth Press, 1–482.

Freud, S. (1917/1963). Mourning and melancholia. In J. Strachey (Ed. & Trans.), *The standard edition of the complete psychological works of Sigmund Freud* (Vol. 14). London: Hogarth Press, 237–260.

Freud, S. (1920/1955). Beyond the pleasure principle. In J. Strachey (Ed. & Trans.), *The standard edition of the complete psychological works of Sigmund Freud* (Vol. 18). London: Hogarth Press, 1–64.

Freud, S. (1926/1959). Inhibitions, symptoms and anxiety. In J. Strachey (Ed. & Trans.), *The standard edition of the complete psychological works of Sigmund Freud* (Vol. 20). London: Hogarth Press, 75–175.

Freud, S. (1940/1964). An outline of psycho-analysis. In J. Strachey (Ed. & Trans.), *The standard edition of the complete psychological works of Sigmund Freud* (Vol. 23). London: Hogarth Press, 139–207.

Geiger, U. (1991). *Reaktionen sechsjähriger Kinder in imaginären Trennungssituationen.* Unpublished dissertation, Institut für Psychologie, Regensburg.

George, C., Kaplan, N., & Main, M. (1985). *The Attachment Interview for Adults.* Unpublished manuscript, University of California, Berkeley.

George, C., Kaplan, N., & Main, M. (1996). *Adult Attachment Interview Protocol* (3rd ed.). Unpublished manuscript, University of California, Berkeley.

Goldberg, S. (1997). Attachment and childhood behavior problems in normal, at-risk, and clinical samples, In L. Atkinson & K. J. Zucker (Eds.), *Attachment and psychopathology.* New York: Guilford Press, 171–195.

Goldberg, S., Corter, C., Lojkasek, M., & Minde, K. (1990). Prediction of behavior problems in four-year-olds born prematurely. *Development and Psychopathology, 2*(1), 15–30.

Goldberg, S., Muir, R., & Kerr, J. (Eds.). (1995). *Attachment theory: Social, developmental, and clinical perspectives.* Hillsdale, NJ: Analytic Press.

Goldberg, S., Perrotta, M., Minde, K., & Corter, C. (1986). Maternal behaviour and attachment in low birth-weight twins and singletons. *Child Development, 57*, 34–46.

Grawe, K. (1998). *Psychologische Therapie.* Göttingen/Bern/Toronto/Seattle: Hogrefe.

Greenberg, M. T., Cicchetti, D., & Cummings, E. M. (Eds.). (1990). *Attachment in the preschool years.* Chicago: University of Chicago Press.

Greenberg, M. T., DeKlyen, M., Endriga, M. C., & Speltz, M. L. (1991). Attachment security in preschoolers with and without externalizing behavior problems: A replication. *Attachment and Developmental Psychopathology, 3*, 413–430.

Greenberg, M. T., DeKlyen, M., Endriga, M. C., & Speltz, M. L. (1997). The role of attachment processes in externalizing psychopathology in young children. In L. Atkinson & K. J. Zucker (Eds.), *Attachment and psychopathology.* New York: Guilford Press, 196–222.

Greenberg, M. T., & Speltz, M. L. (1988). Attachment and the ontogeny of conduct problems. In J. Belsky & T. Nezworski (Eds.), *Clinical implications of attachment.* Hillsdale, NJ: Erlbaum, 177–218.

Greenspan, I., & Lieberman, A. F. (1995a). Current clinical criteria for diagnosing attachment disorders. In J. Belsky & T. Nezworski (Eds.), *Clinical implications of attachment.* Hillsdale, NJ: Erlbaum, 392–394.

Greenspan, I., & Lieberman, A. F. (1995b). The definition and classification of attachment disorders. In J. Belsky & T. Nezworski (Eds.), *Clinical implications of attachment*. Hillsdale, NJ: Erlbaum, 388–390.

Grice, H. P. (1975). Logic and conversation. In P. Cole & J. L. Moran (Eds.), *Syntax and semantics*. New York: Academic Press, 41–58.

Grossmann, K. (1997). *Infant–father attachment relationship: Sensitive challenges during play with toddler is the pivotal feature*. Poster presented at the biennial meeting of the Society for Research in Child Development, Washington, DC.

Grossmann, K., & Fremmer-Bombik, E. (1997). *Longitudinal sequelae of the child–father attachment relationship centering around a play situation*. Paper presented at the 8th European Conference on Developmental Psychology, Rennes, Frankreich.

Grossmann, K., Fremmer-Bombik, E., Rudolph, J., & Grossmann, K. E. (1988). Maternal attachment representations as related to child–mother attachment patterns and maternal sensitivity and acceptance of her infant. In R. A. Hinde & J. Stevenson-Hinde (Eds.), *Relationships within families*. Oxford: Oxford University Press, 241–260.

Grossmann, K., Grossmann, K. E., Spangler, G., Suess, G., & Unzner, L. (1983) Maternal sensitivity and newborns' orientation responses as related to quality of attachment in Northern Germany. In I. Bretherton & E. Waters (Eds.), Growing points of attachment theory and research. *Monographs of the Society for Research in Child Development, 50*(Serial No. 209), 231–256.

Grossmann, K. E. (1988). Longitudinal and systemic-approaches in the study of biological high- and low-risk groups. In M. Rutter (Eds.), *Studies of psycho-social risk: The power of longitudinal data*. New York: Cambridge University Press, 138–157.

Grossmann, K. E. (1993). Bindungsverhalten und Depression. In D. Hell (Ed.), *Ethologie der Depression. Familientherapeutische Möglichkeiten*. Stuttgart/Jena: S. Fischer, 65–79.

Grossmann, K. E., Becker-Stoll, E., Grossmann, K., Kindler, H., Schieche, M., Spangler, G., Wensauer, M., & Zimmermann, P. (1997). Die Bindungstheorie. Modell, entwicklungspsychologische Forschung und Ergebnisse. In H. Keller (Ed.), *Handbuch der Kleinkindforschung* (2nd ed.). Bern: Huber, 51–95.

Grossmann, K. E., Grossmann, K., Loher, I., Scheuerer-Englisch, H., Schildbach, B., Spangler, G., Wensauer, M., & Zimmermann, P. (1993, March 25–28). *The development of attachment and adaption beyond infancy*. Paper presented at the 60th anniversary meeting of the Society for Research in Child Development, New Orleans.

Grossmann, K. E., Grossmann, K., & Zimmermann, P. (1999). A wider view of attachment and exploration: Stability and change during the years of immaturity. In J. Cassidy & P. R. Shaver (Eds.), *Handbook of attachment: Theory, research, and clinical applications*. New York: Guilford Press, 760–786.

Guidano, V. F., & Liotti, G. (1985). A constructivist foundation for cognitive therapy. In M. J. Mahoney & A. Freeman (Eds.), *Cognition and psychotherapy*. New York: Plenum Press, 120–158.

Hansburg, H. G. (1972). *Adolescent separation anxiety: A method for the study of adolescent separation problems*. Springfield, IL: Charles C. Thomas.

Harlow, H. F. (1958). The nature of love. *American Psychologist, 13,* 673–685.

Hartmann, II.-P. (1997a). Mutter-Kind-Behandlung in der Psychiatrie: Eigene Erfahrungen—Behandlungskonzepte und besondere Probleme. *Psychiatrische Praxis, 24,* 172–177,

Hartmann, H.-P. (1997b). Mutter-Kind-Behandlung in der Psychiatrie: Übersicht über bisherige Erfahrungen. *Psychiatrische Praxis, 24,* 56–60.

Henseler, H. (1974). *Narzißtische Krisen. Zur Psychodynamik des Selbstmords.* Reinbek: Rowohlt.

Hesse, E. (1999). The Adult Attachment Interview: Historical and current perspectives. In J. Cassidy & P. R. Shaver (Eds.), *Handbook of attachment: Theory, research, and clinical applications.* New York: Guilford Press, 395–433.

Hock, E., & Schirtzinger, M. B. (1992). Maternal separation anxiety: Its developmental course and relation to maternal mental health. *Child Development, 63,* 93–102.

Hofer, M. A. (1995). Hidden regulators: Implications for a new understanding of attachment, separation, and loss. In S. Goldberg, R. Muir, & J. Kerr (Eds.), *Attachment theory: Social, developmental, and clinical perspectives* (pp. 203–230). Hillsdale, NJ: Analytic Press.

Holmes, J. (1993). *John Bowlby's attachment theory.* London: Routledge.

Holmes, J. (1997). Attachment theory: A biological basis for psychotherapy. *British Journal of Psychiatry, 163,* 430–438.

Hédervári, É. (1995). *Bindung und Trennung. Frühkindliche Bewältigungsstrategien bei kurzen Trennungen von der Mutter.* Wiesbaden: Deutscher Universitäts-Verlag.

Jacobson, E. (1978). *Das Selbst und die Welt der Objekte.* Frankfurt: Suhrkamp.

Jacoby, M. (1998). *Grundformen seelischer Austauschprozesse—Jungsche Therapie und neuere Kleinkindforschung.* Zilrich/Düsseldorf: Walter.

Janus, L. (1996). Schwangerschaft und Geburt aus der Sicht des werdenden Kindes. In E. Brähler & U. Unger (Eds.), *Schwangerschaft, Geburt und der Übergang zur Elternschaft.* Opladen: Westdeutscher Verlag, 90–107.

Kächele, H., Buchheim, A., Schmücker, G., & Brisch, K. H. (2001). Development, attachment and relationship: New psychoanalytic concepts. In F. Henn, N. Sartorius, H. Helmchen, & H. Lauter (Eds.), *Contemporary psychiatry: Vol. 1. Foundations of psychiatry, Part 1: Scientific basis of psychiatry.* Berlin: Springer, 357–370.

Kaplan, N. (1987). *Individual differences in six-year-olds' thoughts about separation: Predicted from attachment to mother at one year of age.* Unpublished doctoral dissertation, University of California at Berkeley.

Klagsbrun, M., & Bowlby, J. (1976). Responses to separation from parents: A clinical test for young children. *British Journal of Projective Psychology, 21,* 7–21.

Klein, M. (1930). The importance of symbol-formation in the development of the ego. *International Journal of Psycho-Analysis, 11*

Klein, M. (1946). Notes on sane schizoid mechanisms. *International Journal of Psycho-Analysis, 27.*

Klein, M. (1983). *Das Seelenleben des Kleinkindes.* Stuttgart: Klett-Cotta.

Köhler, L. (1992). Formen und Folgen früher Bindungserfahrungen. *Forum der Psychoanalyse, 8,* 263–280.

Köhler, L. (1995). Bindungsforschung und Bindungstheorie aus der Sicht der Psychoanalyse. In G. Spangler & P. Zimmermann (Eds.), *Die Bindungstheorie. Grundlagen, Forschung und Anwendung.* Stuttgart: Klett-Cotta, 67–85.

Köhler, L. (1998). Zur Anwendung der Bindungstheorie in der psychoanalytischen Praxis. *Psyche, 52,* 369–403.

Kohut, H. (1971a). *The analysis of the self.* New York: International Universities Press.

Kohut, H. (1971b). Thoughts on narcissism and narcissistic rage. *Psychoanalytic Study of the Child, 27,* 360–400.

Kohut, H. (1977). *The restoration of the self.* New York: International Universities Press.

König, K. (1981). *Angst und Persönlichkeit. Das Konzept vom steuernden Objekt und seine Anwendungen.* Göttingen: Medizinische Psychologie.

Körner, J. (1998). Einfühlung: Über Empathie. *Forum der Psychoanalyse, 14,* 1–17.

Kübler-Ross, E. (1969). *On death and dying.* New York: Macmillan.

Laewen, H.-J., Andres, B., & Hédervári, É. (1990). *Ein Modell für die Eingewöhnungssituation von Kindern in Krippen.* Berlin: FI–Verlag.

Lamott, F., Pfäfflin, F., Ross, Th., Sammet, N., Weber, M., & Frevert, G. (1998). Trauma, Beziehung und Tat. Bindungstheoretische Rekonstruktion interpersonaler Beziehungserfahrungen von Frauen, die getötet haben. *Monatsschrift für Kriminologie und Strafrechtsreform, 81,* 235–245.

Lanczik, M. (1997). "Mother and Baby-Units" an psychiatrischen Krankenhäusern in Großbritannien. *Spektrum, 26,* 38–40.

Laucht, M., Esser, G., & Schmidt, M. H. (1998). Frühe Mutter-Kind-Beziehung: Risiko- und Schutzfaktor für die Entwicklung von Kindern mit organischen und psychosozialen Belastungen: Ergebnisse einer prospektiven Studie von der Geburt bis zum Schulalter. *Vierteljahrszeitschrift für Heilpädagogik und ihre Nachbargebiete, 66,* 1–11.

Lessard, J. C., & Moretti, M. M. (1998). Suicidal ideation in an adolescent clinical sample: Attachment patterns and clinical implications. *Journal of Adolescence, 21*(4), 383–395.

Lichtenberg, J. D. (1989). *Psychoanalysis and motivation.* Hillsdale NJ: Analytic Press.

Lichtenberg, J. D., Lachmann, F. M., & Fosshage, J. L. (1992). *Self and motivational systems: Toward a theory of psychoanalytic technique.* Hillsdale, NY: Analytic Press.

Lieberman, A. F., & Pawl, J. H. (1988). Clinical applications of attachment theory. In J. Belsky & T. Nezworsky (Eds.), *Clinical implications of attachment.* Hillsdale, NJ: Erlbaum, 327–347.

Lieberman, A. F., & Pawl, J. H. (1990). Disorders of attachment and secure base behavior in the second year of life: Conceptual issues and clinical intervention. In M. T. Greenberg, D. Cicchetti, & E. M. Cummings (Eds.), *Attachment in the preschool years.* Chicago: University of Chicago Press, 375–398.

Lieberman, A. F., & Pawl, J. H. (1993). Infant–parent psychotherapy. In C. H.

Zeanah, Jr. (Ed.), *Handbook of infant mental health*. New York: Guilford Press, 427–442.

Lieberman, A. F., & Pawl, J. H. (1995). The treatment of disorders of attachment at the infant–parent program. In J. Belsky & T. Nezworski (Eds.), *Clinical implications of attachment*. Hillsdale, NJ: Erlbaum, 336–346.

Lieberman, A. F., Weston, D. R., & Pawl, J. H. (1991). Preventive intervention and outcome with anxiously attached dyads. *Child Development, 62*, 199–209.

Liotti, G. (1991). Insecure attachment and agoraphobia. In C. M. Parkes, J. Stevenson-Hinde, & P. Marris (Eds.), *Attachment across the life cycle*. London/New York: Tavistock, 216–233.

Liotti, G. (1992). Disorganized/disoriented attachment in the etiology of the dissociative disorders. *Dissociation, 4*, 196–204.

Lorenz, K. (1935). Der Kumpan in der Umwelt des Vogels. *Journal of Ornithology, 83*. English translation 1951 in C. H. Schiller (Ed.), *Instinctive behavior*. New York: International Universities Press, 83–128.

Lorenz, K. (1943). Die angeborenen Formen möglicher Erfahrung. *Zeitschrift für Tierpsychologie, 5*, 235–409.

Lorenz, K. (1935). Der Kumpan in der Umwelt des Vogels. *Journal of Ornithology, 83*. English translation 1951 in C. H. Schiller (Ed.), *Instinctive behavior*. New York: International Universities Press, 83–128.

Lyons-Ruth, K., Alpern, L., & Repacholi, B. (1993). Disorganized infant attachment classification and maternal psychosocial problems as predictors of hostile–aggressive behavior in the preschool classroom. *Child Development, 64*, 572–585.

Lyons-Ruth, K., Connell, D. B., Grunebaum, H. U., & Botein, S. (1990). Infants at social risks: Maternal depression and family support services as mediators of infant development and security of attachment. *Child Development, 61*, 85–91.

Lyons-Ruth, K., Connell, D. B., & Zoll, D. (1989). Patterns of maternal behavior among infants at risk for abuse: Relations with infant attachment behavior and infant development at 12 months of age. In D. Cicchetti & V. Carlson (Eds.), *Child maltreatments*. Cambridge, MA: Harvard University Press, 464–493.

Lyons-Ruth, K., Repacholi, B., McLeod, S., & Silva, E. (1991). Disorganized attachment behavior in infancy: Short-term stability, maternal and infant correlates, and risk-related subtypes. *Attachment and Developmental Psychopathology, 3*, 377–396.

Macey, T. J., Harmon, R. J., & Easterbrooks, M. A. (1987). Impact of premature birth on the development of the infant in the family. *Journal of Consulting and Clinical Psychology, 55*(6), 846–852.

Mahler, M., Pine, F., & Bergman, A. (1978). *The psychological birth of the human infant*. New York: Basic Books.

Main, M. (1981). Avoidance in the service of attachment: A working paper. In K. Immelmann, G. Barlow, L. Petrinovich, & M. Main (Eds.), *Behavioral development: The Bielefeld interdisciplinary project*. New York: Cambridge University Press, 651–693.

Main, M. (1991). Metacognitive knowledge, metacognitive monitoring and singular (coherent) vs. multiple (incoherent) models of attachment. In C. M. Parkes, J.

Stevenson-Hinde, & P. Marris (Eds.), *Attachment across the life cycle*. London/ New York: Tavistock, 127–159.

Main, M. (1995). Recent studies in attachment: Overview, with selected implications for clinical work. In S. Goldberg, R. Muir, & J. Kerr (Eds.), *Attachment theory: Social, developmental, and clinical perspectives*. Hillsdale, NJ: Analytic Press, 407–474.

Main, M., & Cassidy, J. (1988). Categories of response to reunion with the parent at age 6: Predicted from attachment classifications and stable over one-month period. *Developmental Psychology, 24*, 415–426.

Main, M., & Goldwyn, R. (1984). *Adult Attachment Scoring and Classification System*. Unpublished manuscript, University of California, Berkeley.

Main, M., & Hesse, E. (1990). Parents' unresolved traumatic experiences are related to disorganized attachment status: Is frightened and/or frightening parental behavior the linking mechanism? In M. T. Greenberg, D. Cicchetti, & E. M. Cummings (Eds.), *Attachment in the preschool years*. Chicago: University of Chicago Press, 161–182.

Main, M., Kaplan, N., & Cassidy, J. (1985). Security in infancy, childhood and adulthood: A move to the level of representation. In I. Bretherton & E. Waters (Eds.), Growing points of attachment theory and research. *Monographs of the Society for Research in Child Development, 50*(Serial No. 209), 66–106.

Main, M., & Solomon, J. (1986). Discovery of an insecure–disorganized/disoriented attachment pattern. In T. B. Brazelton & M. W. Yogman (Eds.), *Affective development in infancy*. Norwood, NJ: Ablex, 95–124.

Main, M., & Solomon, J. (1990). Procedures for identifying infants as disorganized/ disoriented during the Ainsworth Strange Situation. In M. T. Greenberg, D. Cicchetti, & E. M. Cummings (Eds.), *Attachment in the preschool years*. Chicago: University of Chicago Press, 121–160.

Main, M., & Weston, D. R. (1981). The quality of the toddler's relationship to mother and to father: Related to conflict behavior and the readiness to establish new relationships. *Child Development, 52*, 932–940.

Main, M., & Weston, D. R. (1982). Avoidance of the attachment figure in infancy: Description and interpretation. In C. M. Parkes & J. Stevenson-Hinde (Eds.), *The place of attachment in human behavior*. New York: Basic Books, 31–59.

Mangelsdorf, S. C., McHale, J. L., Plunkett, J. W., Dedrick, C. F., Berlin, M., Meisels, S. J., & Dichtellmiller, M. (1996). Attachment security in very low birth weight infants. *Developmental Psychology, 32*(5), 914–920.

Meyer, A. (1957). *Psychobiology: A science of man*. Springfield: Thoma.

Minde, K. (1993a). Prematurity and serious medical illness in infancy: Implications for development and intervention. In C. H. Zeanah (Ed.), *Handbook of infant mental health*. New York: Guilford Press, 87–105.

Minde, K. (1993b). The social and emotional development of low-birthweight infants and their families up to age four. In S. Friedman & M. Sigman (Eds.), *The psychological development of low-birthweight children*. Norwood, NJ: Ablex, 157–185.

Minde, K. (1995). Bindung und emotionale Probleme bei Kleinkindern: Diagnose und Therapie. In G. Spangler & P. Zimmermann (Eds.), *Die Bindungstheorie. Grundlagen, Forschung und Anwendung*. Stuttgart: Klett-Cotta, 361–374.

Minde, K., Corter, C., & Goldberg, S. (1985). The contribution of twinship and health to early interaction and attachment between premature infants and their mothers. In J. D. Call, E. Galenson, & P. I. Tyson (Eds.), *Frontiers of infant psychiatry.* New York: Basic Books, 160–175.

Murray, L., & Cooper, P. J. (Eds.). (1997). *Postpartum depression and child development.* New York: Guilford Press.

Naslund, B., Persson-Blennow, I., McNeil, T., Kaij, L., & Malmquist-Larsson, A. (1984). Offspring of women with nonorganic psychosis: Infant attachment to the mother at one year of age. *Acta Psychiatrica Scandinavica, 69,* 231–241.

Neumann, E. (1985). *Die Große Mutter: Eine Phänomenologie der weiblichen Gestaltungen des Unbewußten.* Olten: Walter.

NICHD Early Child Care Network. (1994). Child care and child development: The NICHD study of early child care. In L. Friedman & H. C. Haywood (Eds.), *Developmental follow-up: Concepts, domains, and method.* San Diego, CA: Academic Press, 37–396.

NICHD Study of Early Child Care Research Network. (1996, April 20). *Infant child care and attachment security.* Results of the NICHD Symposium, International Conference on Infant Studies, Providence, RI.

Oppenheim, D., Emde, R. N., & Warren, S. (1997). Children's narrative representations of mothers: Their development and associations with child and mother adaptation. *Child Development, 68,* 127–138.

Orlinsky, D. E., Grawe, K., & Parks, B. K. (1994). Process and outcome in psychotherapy—noch einmal. In A. E. Bergin & L. Garfield (Eds.), *Handbook of psychotherapy and behavior change* (4th ed.). New York: Wiley, 270–376.

Papoušek, H. (1977). Die Entwicklung der Lernfähigkeit im Säuglingsalter. In V. H. Braun & A. Hahn (Eds.), *Kultur im Zeitalter der Sozialwissenschaften.* Berlin: Reimer Schriften zur Kultursoziologie, 111–126.

Papoušek, M. (1994). *Vom ersten Schrei zum ersten Wort.* Bern: Huber.

Papoušek, M. (1996). Kommunikations- und Beziehungsdiagnostik im Säuglingsalter—Einführung in den Themenschwerpunkt. *Kindheit und Entwicklung, 5,* 136–139.

Parens, H. (1993a). Does prevention in mental health make sense? In H. Parens & S. Kramer (Eds.), *Prevention in mental health.* Northvale, NJ: Aronson, 105–120.

Parens, H. (1993b). Neuformulierungen der psychoanalytischen Aggressionstheorie und Folgerungen für die klinische Situation. *Forum der Psychoanalyse, 9,* 107–121.

Parens, H. (1993c). Toward the prevention of experience-derived emotional disorders in children by education for parenting. In H. Parens & S. Kramer (Eds.), *Prevention in mental health.* Northvale, NJ: Aronson, 123–148.

Parens, H., & Kramer, S. (Eds.). (1993). *Prevention in mental health.* Northvale, NJ: Aronson.

Parkes, C. M. (1991). Attachment, bonding, and psychiatric problems after bereavement in adult life. In C. M. Parkes, J. Stevenson-Hinde, & P. Marris (Eds.), *Attachment across life cycle* (pp. 268–292). London: Tavistock.

Parkes, C. M., Stevenson-Hinde, J., & Marris, P. (Eds.). (1991). *Attachment across the life cycle.* London/New York: Tavistock.

Pearson, J. L., Cohen, D. A., Cowan, P. A., & Cowan, C. P (1994). Earned- and continuous-security in adult attachment: Relation to depressive symptomatology and parenting style. *Development and Psychopathology, 6*, 359–373.

Pianta, R. C., Egeland, B., & Adam, E. K. (1996). Adult attachment classification and self-reported psychiatric symptomatology as assessed by the Minnesota Multiphasic Personality Inventory?2. *Journal of Consulting and Clinical Psychology, 64*(2), 273–281.

Plunkett, J. W., Klein, T., & Meisels, S. J. (1988). The relationship of preterm infant–mother attachment to stranger sociability at 3 years. *Infant Behavior & Development, 11*(1), 83–96.

Radke-Yarrow, M. (1991). Attachment patterns in children of depressed mothers. In C. M. Parkes, J. Stevenson-Hinde, & P. Marris (Eds.), *Attachment across the life cycle*. London/New York: Tavistock, 115–126.

Radke-Yarrow, M., Cummings, E. M., Kuczynski, L., & Chapman, M. (1985). Patterns of attachment in two- and three-year-olds in normal families and families with parental depression. *Child Development, 56*, 884–893.

Radojevic, M. (1992). *Predicting quality of infant attachment to father at 15 months from prenatal paternal representations of attachment: An Australian contribution.* 25th International Congress of Psychology, Brussels.

Reddemann, L., & Sachsse, U. (1996). Imaginative Psychotherapieverfahren zur Behandlung in der Kindheit traumatisierter Patientinnen und Patienten. *Psychotherapeut, 41*, 169–174.

Reite, M. (1990). Effects of touch on the immune system. In N. Gunzenhauser (Eds.), *Advances in touch: New implications in human development* (Summary Publications in the Johnson & Johnson Pediatric Round Table Series). Skillman, NJ: Johnson & Johnson, 22–31.

Reite, M., & Field, T. (Eds.). (1985). *The psychobiology of attachment and separation.* Orlando, FL: Academic Press.

Remschmidt, H., & Schmidt, M. H. (Eds.). (1994). *Multiaxiales Klassifikationsschema für psychische Störungen des Kindes- und Jugendalters nach ICD-10 der WMO.* Bern: Huber.

Resch, F (1996). *Entwicklungspsychopathologie des Kindes- und Jugendalters.* Weinheim: Psychologie Verlags Union.

Robertson, J. (1952). Film: A two-year-old goes to hospital. London: Tavistock.

Rode, S. S., Chang, P., Nian, P., Fisch, R. O., & Sroufe, L. A. (1981). Attachment patterns of infants separated at birth. *Development Psychology, 17*(2), 188–191.

Rogers, C. (1973). *Die klientenzentrierte Gesprächspsychotherapie.* München: Kindler.

Rogers, S. J., Ozonoff, S., & Maslin-Cole, C. (1991). A comparative study of attachment behavior in young children with autism or other psychiatric disorders. *Journal of the American Medical Association, 30*, 483–488.

Rosenstein, D., & Horowitz, H. A. (1993). *Working models of attachment in psychiatrically hospitalized adolescents: Relation to psychopathology and personality.* Presentation at the Biennial Meeting of the Society for Research in Child Development. New Orleans, LA.

Rudolf, G., Grande, T., & Porsch, U. (1988). Die initiale Patient-Therapeut-

Beziehung als Prädiktor des Behandlungsverlauf. *Zeitschrift für Psychosomatische Medizin und Psychoanalyse, 34*, 32–49.

Rutter, M. (1972). *Maternal deprivation reassessed*. London: Penguin.

Sable, P. (2000). *Attachment and adult psychotherapy*. Northvale, NJ: Jason Aronson.

Sajaniemi, N., Mäkelä, J., Salokorpi, T., von Wendt, L., Hämäläinen, T., & Hakamies-Blomqvist, L. (2001). Cognitive performance and attachment patterns at four years of age in extremely low birth weight infants after early intervention. *European Child and Adolescent Psychiatry, 10*, 122–129.

Sameroff, A. J., & Emde, R. N. (1989). Relationship disturbances in context. In J. Sameroff & R. N. Emde (Eds.), *Relationship disturbances in earl childhood: A developmental approach*. New York: Basic Books, 221–255.

Schain, J. (1989). The new infant research: Some implications for group therapy. *Group, 13*, 112–122.

Scheidt, C. E., Waller, E., Schnock, C., Becker-Stoll, F., Zimmermann, P., Lücking, C. H., & Wirsching, M. (1999). Alexithymia and attachment representation in idiopathic spasmodic torticollis. *Journal of Nervous and Mental Disease, 187*(1), 47–52.

Scheuerer-Englisch, H. (1989). *Das Bild der Vertrauensbeziehung bei 10 jährigen Kindern und ihren Eltern*. Unpublished doctoral dissertation, Regensburg.

Schieche, M., & Spangler, G. (1994). Biobehavioral organization in one-year-olds: Quality of mother–infant-attachment and immunological and adrenocortical regulation. *Pychologische Beiträge, 36*, 30–35.

Schmidt, S., & Strauß, B. (1996). Die Bindungstheorie und ihre Relevanz für die Psychotherapie. *Psychotherapeut, 41*, 139–150.

Schramm, E. (1996). *Interpersonelle Psychotherapie*. Stuttgart/New York: Schattauer.

Schur, M. (1960). Discussion of Dr. John Bowlby's paper. *Psychoanalytic Study of the Child, 15*, 63–84.

Segal, H. (1983). *Melanie Klein. Eine Einführung in ihr Werk*. Frankfurt: S. Fischer.

Slough, N., & Greenberg, M. (1991). Five-year-olds representations of separation from parents: Responses for self and a hypothetical child. In I. Bretherton & M. Watson (Eds.), *Children's perspectives on the family* (pp. 67–84). San Francisco: Jossey-Bass.

Spangler, G. (1998, July 6–7). *Attachment representation and emotional regulation: A psychobiological perspective*. Paper presented at the Development, Structure, and Functioning of Internal Working Models Symposium, Universität Regensburg.

Spangler, G., & Grossmann, K. E. (1993). Biobehavioral organization in securely and insecurely attached infants. *Child Development, 64*, 1439–1450.

Spangler, G., & Schieche, M. (1995). Psychobiologie der Bindung. In G. Spangler & P. Zimmermann (Eds.), *Die Bindungstheorie. Grundlagen, Forschung und Anwendung*. Stuttgart: Klett-Cotta, 297–310.

Spangler, G., & Zimmermann, P. (Eds.). (1995). *Die Bindungstheorie. Grundlagen, Forschung und Anwendung*. Stuttgart: Klett-Cotta.

Sperling, M. B., & Berman, W. H. (Eds.). (1994). *Attachment in adults: Clinical and developmental perspectives*. New York: Guilford Press.

Spieker, J., & Booth, C. L. (1988). Maternal antecedents of attachment quality. In J. Belsky & T. Nezworski (Eds.), *Clinical implications of attachment*. Hillsdale, NJ: Erlbaum, 95–135.

Spitz, R. (1959). *Genetic field theory of ego formation: Its implication for pathology*. New York: International Universities Press.

Spitz, R. A. (1960). Discussion of Dr. John Bowlby's paper. *Psychoanalytic Study of the Child, 15*, 113–117.

Spitz, R. A. (1965). *The first year of life: A psychoanalytic study of normal and deviant development of object relations*. New York: International Universities Press.

Sroufe, L. A. (1979). The coherence of individual development: Early care, attachment and subsequent developmental issues. *American Psychologist, 34*, 84–841.

Sroufe, L. A. (1985). Attachment classification from the perspective of infant–caregiver relationships and infant temperament. *Child Development, 56*, 1–14.

Sroufe, L. A., & Fleeson, J. (1988). The coherence of family relationships. In R. A. Hinde & J. Stevenson-Hinde (Eds.), *Relationships within families: Mutual influences*. Oxford: Clarendon Press, 27–47.

Sroufe, L. A., & Rutter, M. (1984). The domain of developmental psychopathology. *Child Development, 55*, 17–26.

Steele, H., & Steele, M. (1994). Intergenerational patterns of attachment. *Advances in Personal Relationships, 5*, 93–120.

Stern, D. (1986). *The interpersonal world of the infant*. New York: Basic Books.

Stern, D. (1989). The representation of relational patterns: Developmental consideration. In A. J. Sameroff & R. N. Emde (Eds.), *Relationship disturbances in early childhood: A developmental approach*. New York: Basic Books, 52–69.

Stern, D., Sander, L., Nahum, J., Harrison, A., Lyons-Ruth, K., Morgan, A., Bruschweiler-Stern, N., & Tronick, E. (1998). Non-interpretive mechanisms in psychoanalytic therapy: The "somethingmore" than interpretation. *International Journal of Psycho-Analysis, 79*, 903–921.

Stern, D. N., Hofer, L., Haft, W., & Dore, J. (1985). Affect attunement: The sharing of feeling state between mother and infant by means of modal influency. In T. M. Field & N. A. Fox (Eds.), *Social perception in infants*. Norwood, NJ: Ablex, 249–268.

Stevenson-Hinde, J. (1990). Attachment within family systems: An overview. *Infant Mental Health Journal, 11*, 218–227.

Stierlin, H. (1980). *Von der Psychoanalyse zur Familientherapie*. Stuttgart: KlettCotta.

Strauß, B., & Schmidt, S. (1997). Die Bindungstheorie und ihre Relevanz für die Psychotherapie. *Psychotherapeut, 42*, 1–16.

Stuhr, U. (1993). *Die Deutungsarbeit im psychoanalytischen Dialog*. Göttingen: Vandenhoeck & Ruprecht.

Suess, G. J., Grossmann, K. E., & Sroufe, L. A. (1992). Effects of infant attachment to mother and father on quality of adaption in preschool: From dyadic to individual organization of self. *International Journal of Behavioral Development, 15*, 43–65.

Thomä, H., & Kächele, H. (1985). *Lehrbuch der psychoanalytischen Therapie*. Band 1, *Grundlagen*. Berlin/Heidelberg: Springer.

Tinbergen, N. (1952). *Instinktlehre. Vergleichende Erforschung angeborenen Verhaltens.* Berlin/Hamburg: Parey.

Tress, W (1986). *Das Rätsel der seelischen Gesundheit. Traumatische Kindheit und früher Schutz gegen psychogene Störungen.* Göttingen: Vandenhoeck & Ruprecht.

van den Boom, D. C. (1990). Preventive intervention and the quality of mother–infant interaction and infant exploration in irritable infants. In W. Koops, H. Soe, J. van der Linden, P. C. M. Molenaar, & J. J. F Schroots (Eds.), *Developmental psychology behind the dikes.* Delft/Netherlands: Uitgeverij Ekuron, 249–268.

van den Boom, D. C. (1994). The influence of temperament and mothering on attachment and exploration: An experimental manipulation of sensitive responsiveness among lower-class mothers with irritable infants. *Child Development, 65,* 1457–1477.

Van Dijken, S. (1998). *John Bowlby: His early life.* London: Free Association Books.

van IJzendoorn, M. H. (1995a). Adult attachment representations, parental responsiveness and infant attachment: A meta-analysis on the predictive validity of the adult attachment interview. *Psychological Bulletin, 117,* 387–403.

van IJzendoorn, M. H. (1995b). The role of attachment in the development and prevention of sociopathy. *Behavioral and Brain Sciences, 18*(3), 576–577.

van IJzendoorn, M. H., & Bakermans-Kranenburg, M. J. (1996). Attachment representations in mothers, fathers, adolescents and clinical groups: A meta-analytic search for normative data. *Journal of Consulting and Clinical Psychology, 64*(1), 8–21.

van IJzendoorn, M. H., & Bakermans-Kranenburg, M. J. (1997). Intergenerational transmission of attachment: A move to the contextual level. In L. Atkinson & K. J. Zucker (Eds.), *Attachment and psychopathology.* New York: Guilford Press, 135–170.

van IJzendoorn, M. H., & De Wolff, M. (1997). In search of the absent father—meta-analysis of infant–father attachment: A rejoinder to our discussant. *Child Development, 68,* 604–609.

van IJzendoorn, M. H., Frenkel, 0. J., Goldberg, S., & Kroonenberg, P. M. (1992). The relative effects of maternal and child problems on the quality of attachment: A meta-analysis of attachment in clinical samples. *Child Development, 63,* 840–858.

van IJzendoorn, M. H., & Hubbard, F. O. A. (2000). Are infant crying and maternal responsiveness during the first year related to infant–mother attachment at 15 months? *Attachment and Human Development, 2*(3), 371–392.

van IJzendoorn, M. H., Juffer, F., & Duyvesteyn, M. G. C. (1995). Breaking the intergenerational cycle of insecure attachment: A review of the effects of attachment-based interventions on maternal sensitivity and infant security. *Journal of Child Psychology and Psychiatry and Allied Disciplines, 36,* 225–248.

van IJzendoorn, M. H., & Sagi, A. (1999). Cross-cultural patterns of attachment: Universal and contextual dimensions. In J. Cassidy & P. R. Shaver (Eds.), *Handbook of attachment: Theory, research, and clinical applications.* New York: Guilford Press, 713–734.

Vaughn, B. E., & Bost, K. K. (1999). Attachment and temperament. In J. Cassidy &

P. R. Shaver (Eds.), *Handbook of attachment: Theory, research, and clinical applications.* New York: Guilford Press, 198–225.

Wartner, U. G., Grossmann, K., Fremmer-Bombik, E., & Suess, G. (1994). Attachment patterns at age six in South Germany: Predictability from infancy and implications for preschool behavior. *Child Development, 65,* 1014–1027.

Weinfeld, N. S., Sroufe, L. A., Egeland, B., & Carlson, E. A. (1999). The nature of individual differences in infant–caregiver attachment. In J. Cassidy & P. R. Shaver (Eds.), *Handbook of attachment: Theory, research, and clinical applications.* New York: Guilford Press, 68–88.

Werner, E. (1990). Protective factors and individual resilience. In S. Meisels & J. P. Shonkoff (Eds.), *Handbook of early childhood intervention.* New York: Cambridge University Press, 97–116.

Wille, D. E. (1991). Relation of preterm birth with quality of infant-mother-attachment. *Infant Behavior & Development, 14,* 227–240.

Winnicott, D. W. (1958). *Through pediatrics to psychoanalysis.* London: Tavistock.

Winnicott, D. W. (1965). *The maturational processes and the facilitating environment.* New York: International Universities Press.

Wöller, W. (1998). Die Bindung des Mißbrauchsopfers an den Mißbraucher— Beiträge aus der Sicht der Bindungstheorie und der Psychoanalyse. *Psychotherapeut, 43*(2), 117–120.

Zeanah, C. H., & Emde, R. N. (1994). Attachment disorders in infancy and childhood. In M. Rutter, E. Taylor, & L. Hersov (Eds.), *Child and adolescent psychiatry: Modern approaches* (3rd ed.). Oxford: Blackwell Science, 490–504.

Zeanah, C. H., Jr., Mammen, O. K., & Lieberman, A. F (1993). Disorders of attachment. In C. H. Zeanah, Jr. (Eds.), *Handbook of infant mental health.* New York: Guilford Press, 332–349.

Zero to Three/National Center for Clinical Infant Programs. (1994). *Diagnostic classification of mental health and developmental disorders of infancy and early childhood* (DC: 0–3). Arlington, VA: Author.

Zimmermann, P., Spangler, G., Schieche, M., & Becker-Stoll, F (1995). Bindung im Lebenslauf: Determinanten, Kontinuität, Konsequenzen und künftige Perspektiven. In G. Spangler & P. Zimmermann (Eds.), *Die Bindungstheorie. Grundlagen, Forschung und Anwendung.* Stuttgart: Klett-Cotta, 311–332.

# Index

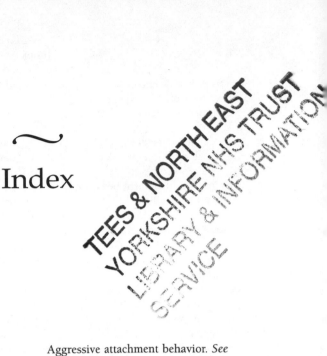